ASYLUM

Memories of a Local Institution

by

Illustrations by David Bucktrout

Memorial Poem by Ronald Ayres

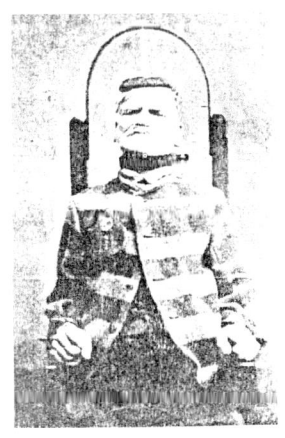

All rights reserved
Copyright Roger Grainger 1996

First published in hardback by Eastmoor Books in 1997, as *'A Place Like That'*
ISBB 0 9528653 0 0

Paperback edition first published by Eastmoor Books in 1997
ISBN 0 9528653 1 9

Re-printed by N. M. Print Services 2014 Tel: 01924 382552

For David and Eleanor Woodcock

A Place Like That
A performing version of 'Asylum' was presented at locations around
Wakefield in 1997 and 1998 by the Pamela Keily Players.

CONTENTS

There's no accounting 7
Historical Note 9
Insiders 11
Prologue 12

LEGACIES
Out of sight, out of mind 22
Therza 23
Don't walk 24
Chained up among the beasts 25
An Official Record 26
For your own and other's safety 27
Clute Ward 28
Get some service in! 29
Gentlemen Only 31
What extreme diseases require 32
Living up to expectations 33
The system and how to play it 34
The Tunnel 35
Roll over 36
On view 37
Housework 38
Safety 39
What absolute power does 41
Taking an interest 42
Cats 43

SURPRISES
Sing it again 46
No place like home 47
For better, for worse 50
Ladies Only 51
Keeping an eye on things 52
I'll just sit here 53
Mary 55
Going with the flow 56
Displaced Persons 57
Cold hands, warm heart 58
Let the trumpets sound 59

Trust 60
Enter then his courts with praise 63
Prayer in a place like that 64
A Christmas carol 65
Tell me about *yourself* 66
Our hospital, our garden 67
Last man in 68
It's better than being bored, love 69
The Sparrow 70

DIRECTIONS
Dramatherapy 74
Annette 76
How should I know? 77
Community Care 78
A place of one's own at last 79
Rest in peace, Ellen 81
Nursing Summer 83
Out on your own 85
No Problem 86
The Semantics of Stigma 88
Looking Back 89

Epilogue 90
R.I.P. 93
1818-1996 by Ronald Ayres 94

INTRODUCTION

by the Earl of Longford

Asylum is a description of a psychiatric hospital of the kind that we would now consider old-fashioned. Until recently there were very many such hospitals in Great Britain. For a short time, more than forty years ago, Roger Grainger was a patient in 'a place like that'. Since becoming an Anglican priest, he has worked mainly in such hospitals. Asylum is the result. In prose and free verse, he lets the hospital speak for itself, describing how it was when he arrived there twenty-five years ago — when the institution still bore the marks of its custodial past — and how it was in the years before it finally closed, quite a different kind of place. The book reflects the love Roger Grainger has for Western Meads (the name has been changed) and the love which, against all the odds, he himself found there. It is a privilege to be allowed to write an introduction to this moving book. I do so with admiration and best wishes for its success.

I would like to thank the following, whose financial support has contributed to the publication of Asylum.

> Les Ablett Esq.
> John Adams Esq.
> The Revd. Malcolm and Mrs. Thelma Aldcroft
> Canon Edward Bailey
> The Revd. Dennis Barraclough
> The Revd. Stanley Baxter
> Peter and Marilyn Billingham
> The Revd. Stuart and Mrs. Susan Brand
> Canon Rex Chapman
> Canon Cyril Dawson
> The Revd. John Ellis
> Mrs. Doreen Grainger
> Michael Grainger Esq.
> The Revd. Geoffrey Hall
> Noel Harrower Esq. and Mrs. Jenny Harrower
> The Rt. Revd. Colin James
> Ms. Marina Jenkyns
> Professor Sue Emmy Jennings
> Ms. Helen Jones
> Mrs. Betty Judge
> The Revd. Simon Parkinson
> Canon Stuart Pearson
> Ms. Andrea Perry
> The Richmond Fellowship
> The Rt. Revd. Barry Rogerson
> The Revd. Colin Shaw
> The Revd. Alastair Shufflebotham
> The Revd. Michael Storey
> The Rt. Revd. Stephen Sykes
> The St. George's Trust
> Wakefield Healthcare
> Benjamin Whitrow Esq.
> Miss Enid Williams
> The Revd. Keith Williams
> A bishop who wishes to remain anonymous
>
> *and*
>
> The District Alliance: In memory of all patients who have used Stanley Royd Hospital.

Lord, you must have felt the lure of places.
There must have been places you knew and loved.
That were special to you.
They wouldn't all have been 'beauty spots'
These places you loved so personally —
It was people you mainly loved, not places —
So some of them must have been unlikely.
Unexpected. Because when it comes down to it,
We love streets more than landscapes, housing
Estates more than forests and mountains.
The beauty of places where people love one another
Is the most precious beauty of all.

So you understand. Lord, how one may love
A place as despised and rejected as this old asylum.
Most people are simply curious, but not that curious —
Their curiosity isn't strong enough to overcome their fear.
Only love can do that

THERE'S NO ACCOUNTING

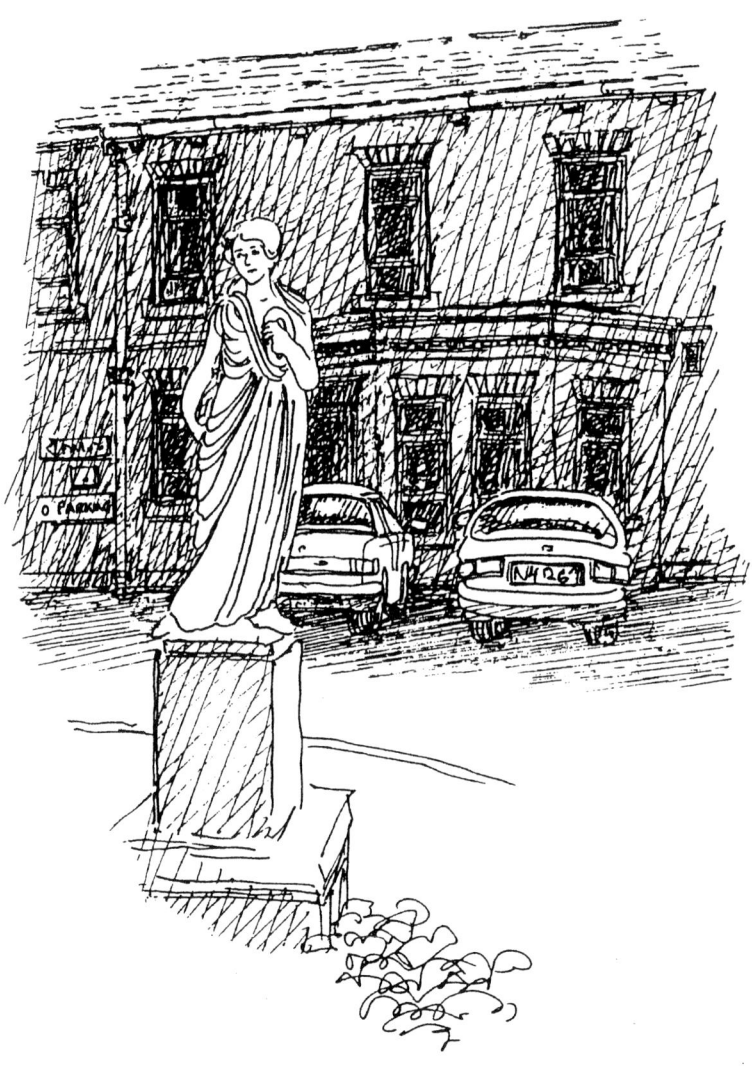

HISTORICAL NOTE

Western Meads is a fictional hospital. This does not stop it having a history, however. It was built in the first decade of the nineteenth century, as part of the first group of the new state psychiatric hospitals inspired by the new Quaker hospital at York. A fine Georgian building, it was meant to accommodate up to one hundred patients, in the hope of restoring as many as possible to the community as soon as this could be managed. The preferred treatment was an early kind of psychotherapy knows as 'moral therapy,' which was based on encouragement and exhortation. It appears to have been remarkably successful, as the discharge rate was as high during the hospital's early years as it was in the nineteen seventies. This, however, did not last. As contemporaries became aware of the usefulness of such places for dealing with individuals who, while they were not actually criminals, would all the same, for one reason or another, be much better 'out of the way,' so the hospital began to grow larger, putting out great stone tentacles, erecting an immense hall and an even larger chapel. The closure of the workhouses in the middle of the nineteenth century resulted in an influx of patients, and the popularity of the 'psychiatric solution' brought the numbers to 3000 by 1937. In 1952 there were more psychiatric admissions in Great Britain than even before, and Western Meads continued to take its share.

In 1959 the Mental Health Act permitted the great majority of patients at Western Meads to become 'informal,' that is, free to leave. Most of those who had been in hospital a long time — a matter of years — preferred to stay. No pressure was put on them to go. The overcrowding which was so much a feature of hospital life was somewhat relieved by those who did go, however, and also by the increased ease of movement inside the hospital now that ward doors had been unlocked. All the same, even in 1975, some dormitories were so overcrowded that patients were sleeping on mattresses down the middle of the room, between the rows of beds.

At this time, and for fifteen years afterwards, the hospital population could be divided into three groups: those who had been mentally disturbed for a long time and were being nursed: those who were permanent residents, but not necessarily ill (or not ill any more): and people who had become, or were in real danger of becoming, mentally ill. These last could expect to be discharged within a matter of months, unless they had nowhere to go — in which case they became members of category two. Owing to the policy of hospital closure ('decarceration') pursued by succesive governments, the number of patients and staff fell dramatically during the last few years and many former patients lived in the local community, mainly in hostels and flats. The majority of these people received psychiatric treatment at home. From time to time many of them came back into hospital for short courses of therapy. Those who remained within the hospital until it formally closed needed perpetual nursing care. About a hundred belonged to category two and simply lived in the hospital, which was reluctant to expel them from the place that had been their home for such a long time. One ward remained, for acutely disturbed patients, admitted on a strictly short-term basis.

Methods of psychiatric treatment had changed over the years. As anti-depressive medication had become more effective, electro-convulsive therapy (ECT) was used less frequently than formerly, and this was widely felt to be a step towards a more 'personal' approach. Doctors were loath to abandon a method of treatment which is sometimes dramatically successful (they are not sure why), but patients often felt that they were being treated as objects rather than as people — particularly when it didn't succeed in removing their depression anyway. In recent years, brain surgery was hardly ever used. There was no formal psychotherapy, but the nurses spent as much time as possible talking and listening to the patients. Visitors had always been rare compared with the general hospital. Those who lived in the town which surrounds Western Meads made nervous jokes about it when they were not simply ignoring its existence. The hospital had a distinguished past and was once famous throughout the country for the skill of its psychiatrists: even during the last twenty years it was the scene of considerable experimentation in the spheres of clinical psychology and rehabilitation of patients, as with many, if not most, hospitals of its kind. However, its reputation within the neighbourhood was almost entirely negative. To people who live in the surrounding area, Western Meads is still 'that place'.

For many this is a place of terror
For a few a place of peace.
But only a few of the many
Have ever been here.

For many it is an idea rather than a place
For a few it is an experience.
Something real, for better or worse.
Part of a life.

Ignorance, however, attracts fear
Like dust collecting on a mantlepiece.
Those who see this place most clearly
Fear it least.

Perhaps this is the principle
On which the hospital has worked until now:
When your understanding isn't knowledge
You're helpless.

INSIDERS

PROLOGUE

This book is about people who, like myself, lived and worked in one of the old mental hospitals. It was very old, having been founded around 1820, and some of these people had been there for a long time. I want to write about them because, for these hospitals, time has run out. They were never popular places; indeed they seem to have been hated and feared by the people who lived round about them, and also, from time to time, by some of the people who lived in them. But not everyone - and not always.

People are often wrong about hospitals like this one. I think that they are blinded by a fear of the unknown which leads them to trust the mind's picture book instead of finding out what is really to be feared; really to be loved. As I went on working at Western Meads Hospital I found more things to be loved, and fewer to be feared. The former were mainly people, the latter almost always the arrangements that people had made, and over which, one way or another, people triumphed.

Love stands out vividly in such a setting; and on reflection Western Meads turns out to have been a pretty vivid place. I didn't always think so, however. I can still remember my first night in the hospital. I had been given a room to myself on the corridor where the doctors on night duty slept. It was a nice little room high up in the old hospital, with a window that looked out over the rooftops. I lay in bed up there, wondering why everything was so quiet. The only thing I could hear was the rattling of the central heating and the soft hum of the doctor's radio from the room next door. I didn't dare go to sleep in case, suddenly, when I wasn't expecting it, somebody shrieked, and I should wake up to the reality of where I was ...

Nobody shrieked of course, that or any night. Never, that is, when I was expecting it. I did quite often hear singing, and sometimes laughter, coming up from the wards. I never found out exactly who was responsible, but I soon realised it was more characteristic of the hospital most of the time than were the occasional cries of distress. When they came they wrenched at the pit of the stomach, pitchforking you into someone else's private hell. When this happened it was best to get down there and see what you could do to help, if anything.

Wherever there is sharing, there is love. The presence of pain and the need to heal and be healed; the exchange of being taking place at the raw edges of life; these are the conditions under which human love is born. In this way, and in this place, these people lived different kinds of lives, discovered different kinds of love. To me, that says as much about the place as it does about them.

It is important to understand that these were all very different kinds of people, very different kinds of lives. It seems to be assumed that a place like that inevitably has the effect of deadening people's individuality, so that everyone becomes the same, saying and doing the same things, speaking and moving in a stereotyped 'patient' way with one or two clearly recognisable variations corresponding to well-known categories of mental illness - the kind of thing you see in TV plays about psychiatric hospitals. It was not like this at all. People's individual differences of character and personality stood out clearly despite the effects of 'institutionalisation', which was more of a protective colouring put on when the occasion demanded than a permanent attitude of mind. I had many lively conversations in the grounds with long-stay residents who seemed not at all bright confronted by the ward duty rota. Be that as it may, a visitor would always find more people here than patients, more variety than sameness. The Meads was more like a village or a small town than a single institution. Perhaps all large institutions are like this. We think of them in terms of a single unitary identity, the special function they perform, which marks them out from the rest of society. To themselves, however, they are their own society, and the attitude of the wider community is just one particular element to be taken into account. To the institution, society itself is one thing among many, often marginalised in precisely the way society marginalises the institution. Obviously it depends on where you stand. In the hospital there is life, variety, interest, friendship, belonging. Or at least there was.

Several reasons were given for the decision to close these hospitals down. First of all, it was stated that changes in the effectiveness of psychiatric treatment made long stays in hospital unnecessary. The new psychoactive drugs rendered the management of psychiatric illness much easier. Now, disturbed patients could be pacified without physical restraint or actual surgery. It became possible to reduce the intensity of the symptoms of mental illness, although it was still not possible to cure it altogether. New non-medical approaches began to be used, with particular success in the treatment of phobias and the rehabilitation of some long-stay patients. It began to look as though it would be possible, by a combination of mood-changing drugs and sophisticated teaching methods, to train patients to earn their own discharge by learning to cope inside the hospital with some of the demands that would be made on them in the world outside the gates.

The second reason concerns society itself. During the 1950s and 1960s there was a growing volume of criticism over the use of psychiatric hospitals as a way of dealing with mental illness. A large amount of sociological research was devoted to examining the pathological effects of institutionalisation. It was argued that these hospitals could not avoid being anti-therapeutic because of the structural rules governing their operation: 'total institutions', they created their own world which had little to do with normality. This was held to be true even if they did not abuse the patients in the ways that everyone believed they did. Living in a place like that carried with it an unavoidable stigma. It was taken for granted that people who lived in an asylum must of necessity be mad. As long as the asylum remained, madness would have little chance of being assimilated into society like all other illnesses. Psychologists and psychiatrists pointed out that the feelings of stigma that prevented patients from having the courage to leave hospital were their own version of society's attitude towards them, for a person's experience of him or herself is affected by his or her own idea of the way he or she is regarded by others. In other words, by putting people into institutions you teach them to see themselves the way they think society sees them - as outcasts, rejects, lunatics. Thus, the problem was believed to be a psychological reaction to a social attitude: if the hospitals were knocked down this would all vanish. Little regard was paid to the existence of actual mental illness, or to the fact that most symptoms occur before anyone has even thought about hospitalisation. On the other hand, there is little doubt that hospitals like this exercised a good deal of their control over patients by manipulating the anti-social tendencies they existed to cure -childish over dependency, self indulgence, the wily ability to 'play the system'.

These are good reasons, but they are not the real reason. The real reason has to be a very good reason; one cannot imagine closing the hospitals down before making alternative provision for either of these reasons, which after all are both therapeutic, at least in the broad sense. The real reason, of course, is money. The origins of the present situation go back a long way. Mental hospitals owe their existence to a particular way of thinking about society, one which says that those who "will not or cannot" work must be carefully segregated from the rest of the community, including those who are capable of working but have been allowed to become a burden on the economy by living off funds provided for poor relief within the community. In its desire to make sure that nobody received support who was not willing to work, a market economy had little time for the Elizabethan Poor Law; if money was to be spent on the poor and the sick, this must happen within special institutions away from the work force. Nowadays the most effective, and the cheapest, way of providing for the health of the work force is by 'community care'. In the nineteenth century the state spent money on social outcasts while the community looked after itself. Nowadays, however, the situation is reversed. Now the community receives state relief and its outcasts must learn to conform.

So far as the state is concerned, they are the wrong people, in the wrong place, at the wrong time, No modern state can afford to spend money on both kinds of people, particularly when the first are profitable and the others are not ... In our own case the mental hospitals are simply left to run down, while attention is concentrated upon kinds of welfare provision which will be available for people living at home. Unfortunately, however, psychiatric help comes far down the list. Ex-psychiatric hospital patients are caught between the devil and the deep blue sea.

During the last ten years local provision for ex-patients has grown from nothing at all to two hostels, a day centre and a drop-in centre run by MIND, open three days a week. There are half a dozen group homes. During this period the hospital population fell by over a thousand people. Some of these have died: but where are the rest? And who cares? The facts speak for themselves. Arguments about improved medicines and the need to liberate men and women from the cruel effects of institutionalisation turn out to be excuses in the light of the unusual determination to empty the buildings and sell them before providing any effective alternative solution. The new drugs were proving much more effective for patients in hospital than they were for people living on their own in the town; they could have been developed as a way of de-institutionalising life on the wards, allowing the hospital to become the kind of community it had always set out to be. Hospitals like this one were criticised for their dehumanising effects from the very beginning - it was only because they appeared to be the cheapest way out of a problem that they were adopted by the government.

Now they are considered to be the dearest way, and so they have to go. In fact, of course, they aren't. The dearest would be proper community provision for the mentally ill. This would involve local clinics, sheltered housing, social centres, a whole range of facilities of a sporting, artistic, recreational kind, where people suffering from mental illness could meet those who weren't. It would also involve extensive schemes for the re-education of the general public, so that a cultural expectation as old as human civilisation can begin to be whittled away, and mentally ill people be received 'into the camp', and fear give way to understanding and sympathy. Perhaps these things are realised by those who are responsible for the closure of the hospitals, and this is why they drag their heels: they are loathe to throw money into a bottomless pit. To do this sort of thing properly would take decades and cost millions of pounds. In the meantime, however, there are the buildings to be sold, some of them on prime industrial sites ...

In a way the situation is favourable towards this kind of attitude. Mentally ill people do not constitute a powerful political lobby. Those who spent years in hospital contributed little or nothing to the national economy;

from that angle their presence will not be missed. They are no longer patients, and can move freely around the country without having to live and work in any one place. They have usually lost touch with any relatives who are still willing to take an interest in them. Very soon, they can drop out of sight altogether. They are really much cheaper than they were when they were in hospital. Some of them are hardly any trouble at all, to the authorities that is, having completely slipped through the community-welfare net. They are sleeping rough and depending on charity, either formal or informal, for whatever food they can lay their hands on. The trouble is still there, of course. It has simply been moved on. It may not still be a financial burden, but it is bound to remain a social and personal one. In hospital the mentally ill were looked after by professionals. Wherever they are now, with their relatives at home or among strangers in the church crypt, they are almost certainly at the centre of disturbance.

Now, however, it is an unofficial disturbance, one that the government can ignore but others can't. It is not only fear, terror of the unknown and seemingly unknowable, that drives people away from mental illness; it is also experience, the knowledge that one has tried and tried, and failed to make any impression, to relieve the pain to any significant degree at all. Some kinds of mental illness - most kinds at some times - need to be contained, to be held gently but strongly until the crisis is past. This is what makes me feel so sad when I think of those who have slipped below even the charity line and are now totally alone. How many men and women camp out in the corridors of condemned buildings and long to be in hospital? How many of them remember Western Meads? I'm glad that most of my friends died before this could happen to them.

The last years of Western Meads' life were not all gloom and despair, which makes the eventual closure of the hospital seem sadder than ever. The fact is, however much effort is put into providing the statutory benefits presented in successive Mental Health Acts, life can be less tolerable outside the hospital than inside. Community care can turn out to be cold comfort for those who have known the family atmosphere of the hospital. The new kinds of treatments made Western Meads far less custodial in its attitudes towards the patients. There were now more opportunities for choice in their daily lives, and the subject of discharge, hardly ever mentioned in the long and medium-stay wards when I first arrived, became a favourite topic. Would it be better outside? How will I cope? Do I have to go? People started to spend more time window-shopping in the town, or visiting friends and relatives. Rehabilitation became the principal focus of everything that happened, and a great deal of effort went into finding out the kinds of environment individuals would like to live in when they were discharged from hospital.

This concentration upon the patients as people, with particular likes and dislikes, brought new life to the hospital as a whole; up to now it had happened in some wards, not in others. Now there were more discussion groups, more individual counselling sessions. Some of the approaches were quite new: after all it was a new situation we were preparing for and required a new approach. For instance, we ended up with eight clinical psychologists instead of the solitary practitioner in post when I arrived. If patients who had been in hospital for thirty years were to survive, there was a good deal of teaching and learning to be done. Clinical psychologists and occupational therapists worked hard in order to widen patients' awareness of themselves as people involved in a wider world of relationships than that of the hospital ward, or even the hospital itself. Their allies in this were the creative therapists (art and drama), aiming at the kind of acceptance of self that had never been contemplated before in a place like this.

Relaxation of the rules that have defined its institutional presence so rigidly for so long, coupled with a change in philosophy towards personal growth and self expression, made the Meads an interesting place to work in during these latter years. I believe it was a good place, too, for people suffering from mental illness, because it combined security and hope in ways that it had never been able to do before. At this point, when it seemed to be approaching the position of a therapeutic community for the first time in its existence, the hospital surrendered to the pressure of official policy and began to make definite plans to close down. Out of 36 wards and departments, two wards would be kept open but they would function as the Acute Unit of the Psychiatric Department of the general hospital. Western Meads itself, the old hospital, was no more.

It is not difficult to guess who the victims are. It is always the same ones. Those who were locked in when they need not have been are the same ones that were kicked out when they should not have been. Those are the ones who suffer. Decisions like this are taken at a different level from that at which life is actually lived - the life of those affected, that is. Once taken, they must be carried out. What may seem reasonable in a White Paper can cover over a universe of pain. The trouble with decisions which don't personally affect the makers is that they tend to be extreme. If you yourself are involved you can usually see good in both sides of the question; if you are not, you tend to favour 'going the whole hog'.

Certainly, with regard to psychiatric hospitals there has been little question of compromise.. Patients have been expelled or incarcerated, locked in or left in danger of homelessness. Those who defend this point out that every official decision is bound to cause someone hardship. Growth inevitably involves suffering, yet people survive. It doesn't do to offer people too much help, as it undermines their own determination to do their best. Besides, you could say anything, anything at all, is better than living in a place like that ...

I don't agree. And I know others who don't as well. But I no longer know exactly where they are ... Those who were patients are now ex-patients - if they are still alive. Nowadays the people in this book, or people like them, are living in the local neighbourhood, only a few miles away from the place where they spent so many years as patients. Some, however, have been sent back to the areas in which they were born and from which they originally came to Western Meads. It's hard to tell which is worse: life among those who don't know who you are or where you come from, or among those who know all too well. Or think that they do.

The presence among them of former patients of the hospital seems to have had a mixed effect on the local residents. Confronted by the difference between real people and the cultural stereotype of mental illness, most people have adapted well to the new situation. One or two have made nostalgic remarks to the effect that, maybe, Western Meads wasn't such a bad place after all, or not as bad as they used to think. They go on to say that at least people weren't lonely there, and the staff seem to have been kind. They seem to be saying this because they are genuinely sympathetic towards ex-patients, and not simply because they themselves feel safer as far away from mental illness as it is possible to get.

This, of course, is how they do feel. Even those who deplored the old mental hospitals and longed for their closure are alarmed by a situation in which there is so little medically supervised provision for people suffering from mental illness. This seems to me to be a problem of national importance. As I have written elsewhere, people are conscious of having been "required to take part, along with the rest of society, in an intensive social revolution". They are aware that the revolution is far from over, and will not be until a way has been found of taking account of mental illness which neither regards it as an unspeakable evil which deprives its sufferers of the love and respect due to them as human beings, nor pretends that it does not really exist at all, being simply a matter of social adjustment which has been exaggerated out of all proportion by successive attempts at finding a solution. The people I have spoken to feel that the problem remains wholly unsolved by simply closing down mental hospitals and leaving the mentally ill to find their own level within the local community (with some help, of course, from various kinds of health professionals).

Mental illness has always been a problem for society as a whole as well as for the individuals and families most closely concerned. Over the ages, different ways of coping with it have been tried, none of them very successfully, and all of them involving the invention of a special social category for the insane in order to separate them from other kinds of people, including people who are physically sick or disabled. The system of incarceration in large mental hospitals was both expensive, and ergonomically wasteful, creating illness as well as relieving it. From this point of view, the cure itself needed radical surgery.

The wound will take a long time to heal. As I write this, Western Meads is in the process of finally closing its doors. A deadline has been set for the summer of next year. There are still two hundred patients in the hospital; when I joined the staff as Chaplain twenty years ago there were sixteen hundred. It has taken many months to get even this far, and this last stage is the most difficult of all. The patients who are still here are the ones who didn't want to leave, and those whom the hospital was least willing to part with. In other words, the most determined and the most dependent. Responsibility for making provision for remaining patients is divided between the Community Trust - the successor to the old Hospital Management Committee - and the District Health Authority. The first body has charge over patients who are considered to be still in need of specifically psychiatric care, while the Health Authority is responsible for those who are no longer in need of psychiatric treatment and are to be discharged altogether from the care of the National Health Service, in some cases after many years. Both the Trust and the Authority are pushing forward their plans to make the necessary provision before next summer's deadline. The Trust concerns itself with an assessment unit and day hospital for elderly patients, a residential home for 'persons with complex needs suffering regularly from high levels of psychiatric disability', two homes for younger rehabilitation patients and three 'community units for the elderly', as well as a new day hospital for patients who are not ill enough to warrant their being admitted to the one remaining acute psychiatric ward. The Authority concentrates on a range of facilities for patients 'defined as primarily in need of social care, and those who are frail and elderly'. The local Department of Social Services is also heavily involved in the provision of services.

The number of agencies involved, and the difficulty of deciding who is financially responsible for what has resulted in a long period of confusion, during which time those patients who were able to leave hospital under their own steam have been settling in to their new lives, in hostels, group homes or flats. Significantly enough, part of the delay in finally closing the hospital down has been caused by the protective attitude Western Meads seems always to have had towards its patients: "The hospital will not close down until everybody has a place to go to." In fact, only when it does finally close will the last patient leave. Until then she simply refuses to be moved from the place that for the last sixty years has been her home.

LEGACIES

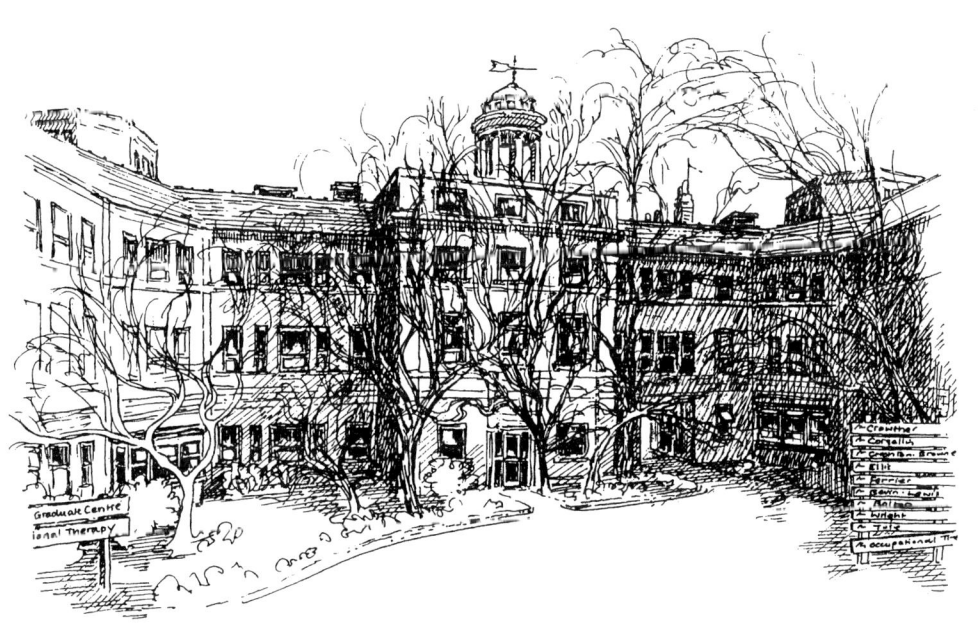

The hospital stands on high ground at the city edge.
Black local stone, extended like a fortress
Tower and chimney part of the familiar skyline
and yet a world away, beyond the pale in fact-
A homely reminder of the unthinkable,
Spectre at the elbow, unacknowledged terror, childhood
Nightmare, Western Meads. You'd better
Behave yourself or you'll find that's where you are ...
The Meads. Certainly sounds harmless, but then that
Is intentional. They wanted a nice name, and who
Can blame them; but whatever it does for them
It certainly terrifies the rest of us. People who go there,
and return to talk to us about it, say it's not really so bad,
Say that there are worse places. It may be so, certainly:
On balance, we'd rather not know.

OUT OF SIGHT, OUT OF MIND

When Therza died I inherited some of her photographs. She used to carry them round in her capacious old handbag, and sometimes she would take them out and show them to people she approved of, which wasn't everybody by any means. She was eighty when she died, in 1980, and there seemed to be no living relatives. So I kept a hold on her photos. I don't think she would have minded, as we always got along pretty well together and no-one else showed any interest. Actually, they were fascinating photographs, not because of their quality as reproductions or the artistic skill they showed, but because of their subject matter. They were all at least sixty years old and showed people, mainly nurses, who had worked at the hospital in the 1920s, when Therza was a young woman patient. One of them shows Therza herself, in a flowered dress, holding on a large hat. It was taken in the hospital grounds during a patients' cricket match. The spectators' dress has changed a lot but the players look much the same as always, only a bit smarter. There are some snaps of nurses in uniform; one of two young nurses, perhaps ward maids, pushing each other over on the lawn and roaring with laughter. The picture I love most, however, is of a ward sitting room. This may be a little earlier than 1920 - it looks mid-Victorian but almost certainly belongs to this century. Two nurses in white lace caps, long white aprons covering their voluminous black skirts, are shown standing in front of a black mahogany sideboard. This is covered with shining silver ornaments, including several pictures in silver frames. What appears to be a Georgian teapot and sugar sprinkler are at one end of the sideboard and an ornate silver table lamp at the other. On each side is an armchair, with a crocheted antimacassar and an embroidered cushion. Unfortunately, you can't see the colour of the embroidery but the cushions themselves, like the antimacassar, are in white. On the wall behind are Victorian mountain landscapes and two ordinary gas lamps.

THERZA

Just inside the iron railings,
Marking out the shape of the whole place,
A shallow ditch runs round. The grass
Grows wild. It's not a path,
More of a gesture.
A sign which says keep out
More clearly than the railings.
Keep Out. Don't Walk.
Wherever you stand, which way you look,
Don't walk ...
Not here.

DON'T WALK ...

When the cellar floor of the old building was taken up some years ago, it revealed a long stone pavement sloping inwards from either wall to form a narrow gutter, leading to a drain half way along the corridor. This, it seems, represented the unacceptable underside of late eighteenth century moralising. This part of the hospital was for the people who couldn't be argued or exhorted out of their madness, and so were better regarded simply as animals. Men and women were kept locked up in narrow cells, each with a cubicle alongside to house the servant employed as their custodian, who acted as nurse, jailor and - quite literally - groom or stable boy. It was here that the prisoner-patients were chained up at weekends while the warder-attendants enjoyed a few hours rest and relaxation, no doubt well-deserved. Straw was provided for them to sit or lie down, to the extent that their shackles allowed them to do so, and loaves of bread and dishes of porridge were left within their reach, while the gutters provided what was necessary for relieving their other natural functions. On their return, their attendants mucked out by swilling water down the central sluice and scrubbing the length of the corridor with long-handled brooms ...

For much of the hospital's life this cellar floor was covered over, to look like the corridors in the three floors above. About twenty years ago, round about the time that the hospital museum first opened, the boards were taken up and the hospital invited to take a look at its own history. Soon after it was covered up again, so that all you can see now are the iron staples in the walls that took the chains.

CHAINED UP AMONG THE BEASTS

Some of the exhibits here would turn your blood cold.
Mind you, that's true of most medical museums -
You have to be cruel to be kind.
(You not me - I don't want anything to do with this.)
There are cast iron baths for steaming madness out
Or freezing it in; revolving chairs for changing your outlook and
Inducing a new look at life; carefully constructed
Strait jackets; devices for electrocuting the brain.
Worst of all, even worse than the harmless looking black boxes
And the narrow knives, are the opinions of the doctors themselves,
The reasons why people are to be considered insane,
The kinds of behaviour that are always signs of madness,
The circumstances which indicate these kinds of intervention.
Everything has been superbly laid out,
Reflecting a high degree of skill and not a little
Personal devotion. After all, it can only be seen
As extremely instructive.

AN OFFICIAL RECORD ...

Before the 1959 Mental Health Act, many wards were kept locked in order to prevent patients from gaining their freedom, and the grounds were surrounded by iron railings to a height of eight feet or more. The entire hospital was organised along lines of total patient security, and special 'airing courts' were provided, corresponding to the exercise yards of prisons. Even after the Act, some parts of the building were still kept locked, for the containment of 'difficult or recalcitrant' patients. This went on for the next thirty years; first of all an entire landing - four wards - was kept secure, and then a pair of wards, one male and one female. When the time came for the hospital to close, there was still one locked ward. By this time, however, the new Regional Secure Units had taken over this particular role, and the locked ward was used only for times when patients needed 'special care' (the hospital's term for increased supervision). These were usually men and women who had lived in the hospital on a permanent or semi-permanent basis for years rather than months. A period of special care was considered to be the best way of dealing with outbreaks of violence or sustained aggression, even though the tremendous improvement in psychiatric drug therapy had rendered incarceration unnecessary. In the circumstances, patients were confirmed in their interpretation of the situation with regard to the locked wards. Their worst fears were confirmed. They were places of punishment, the inevitable consequence of what the hospital saw as disobedient behaviour. They had come into hospital because they were sick and needed medical help. The hospital itself, however, saw them rather differently from the psychiatrist; sick behaviour was simply bad, wicked, disobedient; and if you indulged in it you would surely end up where you deserved to be - 'on Ward Seven'. It was a terrifying idea and in light of the circumstances, a deeply confusing one. As long as treatment was identified institutionally with punishment, hospitals like this one contributed to the image of madness as a condition of intractable unreason, in respect of which no person and no place could be trusted.

I've known Clute Ward for twenty years
- Longer than some of the patients there.
It's not a ward to stay long on -
Just long enough.

People have tried to brighten it up
- Curtains, easy chairs, one of those sideboards with glass in,
Even a few small china animals.
But it's no use.

The hospital seems to need a place like this
To accommodate what it can't contain:
Clute is useful for being what it is
A dump.

For twenty years it has housed people who don't fit,
People who don't even fit here.
Those who have had to be put away
Twice over.

Through 'successive changes in hospital policy'
It's been consistent rejection, inflexible contempt
For everyone, old or young, docile or disturbed,
Living (or dying) on Clute.

CLUTE WARD

Frank had spent over twenty years in various mental hospitals up and down the northern part of England. He liked to tell fellow patients about the differences between them from a patient's point of view - the advantages of Rainhill over Parkside, or De La Pole over Prestwich, the strange cultural variations of hospital procedure between institutions in different counties, the unique terrors of Rampton itself. Frank was a professional, a specialist in the weirdly fascinating mixture of science and sadism, medical expertise and crass institutional manipulation and repression of the human spirit which constitutes the lore of mental hospitals, the cherished tradition of the psychiatrically stigmatised. Frank had penetrated the barrier which divides the people who have known the joys and terrors of the insane asylum from everyone else in the world who can only look on in ashamed fascination. It was his duty and privilege - and above all his satisfaction - to initiate them into his world. It was not enough just to be a mental patient; you had to learn how to think like one, how to see yourself and the rest of the world from that unique point of view. For this you needed a teacher. This was the task that Frank had undertaken to perform, and he did it with complete devotion, and also a good deal of skill.

Frank's message concerned the inmates of mental hospitals, most of whom, Frank maintained, were obviously sane. He provided evidence for this by quoting the cases of a whole string of patients whom he had known personally over the years, who by their behaviour and the things that they said were completely normal. Some of these people were decidedly above average, in fact. "There was this bloke at High Royds who taught himself German in six months by one of those correspondence courses. I'm not kidding - there was a German doctor there, he's most likely still there. He thought he was a German, used to talk to him in German", or "You should have seen old Pete! He was amazing; he'd got the whole ward organised like a bookie's office, putting bets on for all the staff. He even had a bloke with a typewriter to do his secretarial work for him." "Where did he get a secretary from, Frank?" "Where d'you think? Another patient used to be an accountant. Came in very useful for keeping the books! No mucking about, though, you couldn't get anything past Pete ..." You couldn't get much beyond Frank either, for that matter.

GET SOME SERVICE IN!

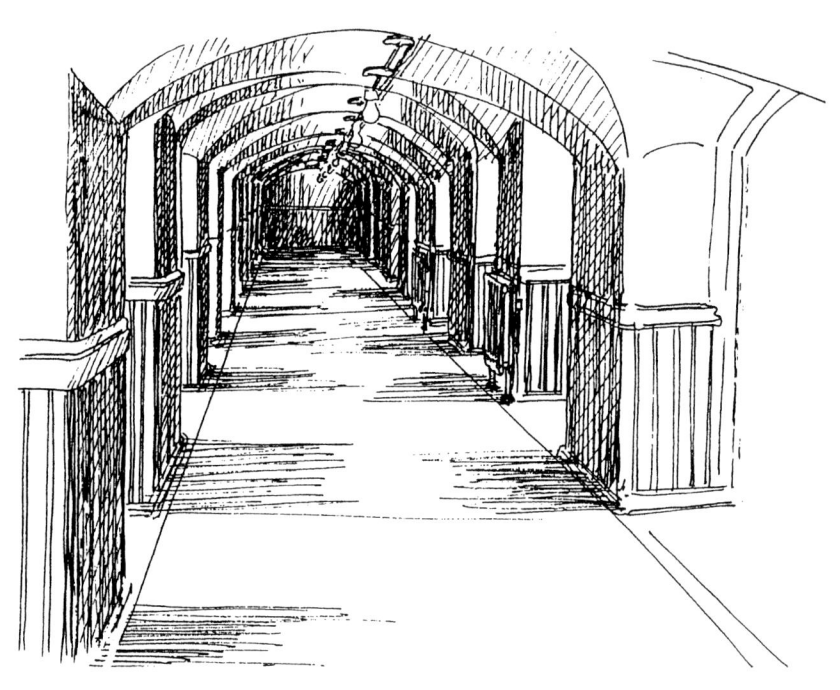

This is the oldest part of the hospital. Ssh, go quietly,
It's half past one, and there's no-one around. The residents are having their afternoon nap.
The atmosphere is heavy with pipe tobacco and floor polish.
Here
The vaulted corridors meet to make a circle round the central column, the spindle-tree of the hospital.
Although the space is open it still feels shut in -
We're several yards from the nearest window. Meanwhile, the faint noise of snoring
Enters from the sitting room. Here, in arm chairs ranged along the walls,
A dozen old men have taken shelter and are now fast asleep,
Their legs reaching outwards to each other in a gesture of mutual support and
Affirmation. The corridor is like a tunnel, leading to the central space,
The world's navel, institutional omphalos,
This is just the sitting room, halfway between station waiting room
And a London club. It's the kind of thing
You could see anywhere. Come on,
We'll find some fresh air. We don't want them to wake up
And see us looking down on them.

GENTLEMEN ONLY

In the nineteen fifties, hospitals like this one still used a treatment called 'Deep Insulin Therapy'. As the locked doors and iron grille confined patients to a particular place, so the deep insulin treatment kept them imprisoned in an endless present. On Bollington Ward patients passed their days islanded by nightmare, separated from past and future by a seemingly endless succession of insulin comas. 'Deep Insulin' was a kind of chemical shock treatment. Patients were given enough insulin to send them into a coma, and then their blood sugar level was brought rapidly back to normal, bringing them back to consciousness again. Put like that, the process does not sound particularly alarming. In fact, it was extremely, even brutally uncomfortable. Going into the coma was painless: the nightmare came when they were coming out. This process of struggling back into life was terrifying. Patients screamed and shouted for help, lashing about, kicking the wooden sides of their cots until their legs and feet bled. The struggle for consciousness was like trying to run from a blazing car with legs that have had the bones taken out of them, or pulling yourself out of the deep end of a swimming bath when you can't swim and they're holding out a pole covered with grease ... Only this was your brain that it was all happening to and you couldn't think what to do because you couldn't think ...

On Bollington Ward patients never had an opportunity to speak to a doctor and ask him how such treatment could possibly help them. Now and again, once a fortnight or so, an assistant psychiatrist used to walk through the ward, but he didn't stop. As soon as he appeared in the doorway a group of patients would rush up to him: he would ignore them. How treatments worked, even whether or not they worked, was his business not theirs. "When will I be able to go home, Doctor?" - "Have I nearly finished my treatment?" - "Can I speak to you for a moment, Doctor, I haven't managed to speak to anyone since I came." The doctor went out, just as he had come in, without a word.

WHAT EXTREME DISEASES REQUIRE

In a padded cell there's little you can do
Because what you can do, or start doing,
Doesn't count. Doesn't really get you anywhere.
It's as if you can't make any impact, anywhere,
On anything.
This is a familiar feeling, but never so much as in here,
In a machine for stopping you.
You're in it, it's built round you, and it's waiting
For you to start.
Maybe you could do something, make your mark
On this vinyl and canvas, these white painted hinges,
But it would be expecting it. It's so clean, this,
It's dirty.
It's got dirt in mind. Your dirt. You've been shut
In your own shit. How
Encouraging.

LIVING UP TO EXPECTATIONS

People like Jimmy carry a hospital around with them. To be saddled with a psychiatric diagnosis is to be shut up inside a social stereotype - always to be one kind of person because nobody will ever see you as anything different. You wear your 'illness' everywhere you go, like a scuba-diver's wetsuit. You can imagine how limiting this is - particularly as the kind of person you are stuck with is never the kind you want to be, or the kind you know you can be. Who would want to be known by his or her mental illness? And yet that's precisely what a lot of people are known by.

Jimmy used to wander along by the perimeter fence round the hospital, talking to anyone he could find about railways. On one occasion this was myself. He had been an engine driver on the 'Lanky', the old Lancashire & Yorkshire Railway. I have always been fascinated by steam railways, ever since I used to collect engine numbers as a kid, but I hadn't met many actual drivers, so Jimmy's stories filled me with delight. Here at last was someone who was able to explain how the valve gear worked. "Course I will," he said. "We'll need some paper." And away he started across the playing fields towards the wing of the hospital he was living in, with me walking beside him. When he reached his ward the Charge Nurse beckoned me on one side and asked me politely if Jimmy talked to me. I said he did, quite a lot and quite often. "That's interesting," said the Charge Nurse. "He never says a word when he's on the ward." I asked him how long Jimmy had been in hospital. I said that Jimmy had told me it was twenty-seven years. "Oh, he said that did he? I shouldn't pay much attention to him. He's schizophrenic, you know." Jimmy hobbled into the ward office and stood waiting for his tablets. I looked at him again. Somehow he looked quite different. I said, "All right, Jimmy?" He grinned and shuffled away.

THE SYSTEM AND HOW TO PLAY IT ...

At one end plumbers, electricians, carpenters,
Shoemakers, tailors, the upholsterer's shop,
At the other the trees, a steep green slope,
The open sky. Between, for fifty yards
The tunnel. It's a real tunnel, not just a passage,
Wide enough to handle a tube train
Long enough too, if you're looking from this end.

Nothing travels along the tunnel except cats
And different kinds of cable, pipe and conduit -
electricity, gas and water; sewage and central heating -
Clinging close together for mutual support,
Gleaming dully along the vault's length. The longer
It stretches, the darker the tunnel gets; so that at the end
Even daylight fights for survival. It's no good

I can't possibly make it that far.

THE TUNNEL

The original hospital was a small compact building designed to hold fifty patents. Soon afterwards it began to expand until, by 1930, it contained three thousand souls. The actual building had stopped growing by nineteen hundred, however. During the early years of the century it was a case of squeezing up to find room. Some people came to Western Meads because they were identifiably ill; many more because there was nowhere else for them to go. It was a place for people to go whom other people found hard to live with but who were not actually criminals; people who were considered to be lazy, or quarrelsome, or to have anti-social habits. The records preserved in the hospital museum list patients admitted for 'having an illegitimate child', 'frequenting theatres', or even 'reading books and novels'. When the workhouses set up by the Elizabethan Poor Law were closed down, ex-residents turned to the local asylum as the only available place of shelter. After all, you didn't need to be very mad. You didn't need to be very mad in the forties and fifties of this century either; it was a time when adolescent identity crisis was almost synonymous with incipient schizophrenia, and there were proportionately more admissions in 1952 than any other year, before or since. The hospital continued to take everything (and everyone) that was thrown at it, squeezing beds into corners and down the middle of wards, adapting sitting rooms into make-shift dining areas, filling the airing courts with 'temporary' wooden buildings until the stone rind of the hospital began to swell like an overripe cheese.

ROLL OVER ...

People who belong to important professions
(Anyone who isn't a patient, in fact)
Are invited to come to the Friday Social.
If you come, you meet the Hospital Administrator
And shake hands with Clinical Psychologists
And some psychiatrists.

Even if you are not a professional
You are not excluded! Even patients
Are not entirely shut out from this event,
But may look down on the gathering from above
Where on all four sides the open gallery has been glassed in for reasons of safety.
It is a splendid viewpoint for the non-professionals,
Who can sometimes look just as interesting and colourful
In their pyjamas and nightdresses, their hospital blue and red dressing gowns,
As the folk they have come to gaze at.
While at the same time only in a restricted sense
Crowding the gods.

ON VIEW

In the old days, before we had the huge electric polishers, the patients used to polish the floors themselves. This involved working away for hours on end with an instrument known as a 'bumper', which resembled a broom with an extra-large handle and a heavy, cylindrical block of wood fixed on the end in place of the broom-head, and a piece of cloth soaked in liquid floor-polish wrapped round it. You couldn't just pick it up and start polishing with it. You had to learn how to use it, and this wasn't easy because it meant swinging the whole contraption from your left hand to your right hand and back again while turning round in a wide circle, so that first one arm and then the other was almost dragged from its socket by the weight of the bumper's head striking the floor. Left, right, left, right; even at this distance in time my arms ache to think about it. The slide, bang and slide of the bumper, the smell of institutional polish, the diamonds of sunlight cast on the parquet floor by the iron grille which shut us in from the airing court while presenting a view of open grounds and flower beds beyond - "Go on, don't slacken off just because my back's turned! It's your ward - Make it shine like the sun!"

HOUSEWORK

This place is huge. It's more immense
Than any sum of parts, as exhaustive as imagination.
I hug its lovely vastness to myself
And feel it pressing me together - No chance here
Of getting lost. Where you can distinguish landmarks
That's where you get lost.

This place is bigger than I thought it was. It's wider
Than my thinking, like my feeling.
It goes on forever, growing more intense, more authentic.
I see myself running from ward to ward, screaming,
Cannoning from corner to corner, breaking down doors,
Careering to the centre, and the centre's centre.
Screaming.

Maybe tomorrow. Meanwhile this place is huge -
And it's me.

SAFETY

Kent Ward is what used to be called an 'admission ward'. This was rather a misleading term, because it seemed to suggest that the ward represented a kind of introductory phase of being a patient, and that one might expect to move on into other wards during one's stay in Western Meads, which was not necessarily - or even usually - the case. In fact, admission wards were small psychiatric hospitals on their own, as it were, distinguished from other wards because their patients were considered to be more or less easily diagnosable and treatable, and consequently returnable to their homes and families. There were only five or six admission wards. The great majority of wards were for patients who might, for one reason or another, be expected to stay longer in hospital; people whose illness or disability would take longer to treat, if it could indeed be medically treated at all; those whose normal environment was thought to contribute to their illness; those who had no home to go to and were consequently better off in the hospital; those who just lived there, and for whom the hospital itself was home.

Admission wards, then, were mainly for 'short-stay' patients and the rest of the hospital for 'long-stay' ones. By itself, apart from the immense main block at Western Meads, Kent Ward would have seemed an extremely large building. It had been built at the beginning of this century, to have forty patients - almost as many, that is, as the original main hospital. The dining and sitting rooms were on the ground floor, together with the Electro-Convulsive Therapy Treatment Room. Upstairs were the dormitories for men and women, and a few small rooms which could be locked from the outside but not the inside. These were used for patients whom it was thought necessary to 'restrain'. Upstairs, too, was the consultant psychiatrist's office, and the large sitting room in which he held his 'ward rounds'. In some admission units these rounds involved walking round and talking to patients. In others they consisted of a more or less formal lecture delivered by the consultant to his team of sister, nurses, occupational therapist and perhaps a psychologist, of precisely what was wrong with particular patients and how they were to be regarded, and consequently treated.

The consultant over Kent Ward was, for many years, a neuro-psychologist as well as a psychiatrist, and tended to be more interested in candidates for brain surgery than other kinds of patients, whom he regarded as probable malingerers. Reflecting the personality of the consultant-in-charge, the regime in each admission ward was almost completely different from the others. No-one else thought like Dr O'Keefe on this matter, but in his own domain his thinking went unquestioned. At the level of actual diagnosis and treatment of acute cases, the Meads might as well have been five or six separate hospitals. The only one left now is Kent, which forms part of the General Hospital. Dr O'Keefe, however, passed from the scene many years ago.

This is Sister McDermot: "Psychiatric nursing
Is entirely different from nursing in a general
Hospital. We try to take a personal interest
In all our patients. We spend more time
With them. And we always try, so far as we can,
To answer their questions. After all,
They are people, not just patients -
They are people like us."

This is SEN Cartwright, in charge of this landing.
If you ask her nicely, or even if you don't,
She will show you the punishment cells. "Look
At this huge brass mortice lock and the tiny inspection window.
Please feel the weight of this door, solid wood. All, happily,
Now in the past! But please remember - "
The State Enrolled Nurse pauses: what she remembers
She'd rather not say,

TAKING AN INTEREST ...

There seem to have been cats everywhere. If you wander through the wards where the elderly women patients used to live, you will find pictures of cats stuck up all over the place, on locker doors, notice boards, walls, so that you begin to imagine you've found your way into an Egyptian tomb. Real cats were not allowed on the wards - not officially permitted. Hence the presence of so many pictures, glossy greeting-card icons, faded cuttings from magazines, crayon drawings done by great nieces and nurses' children. I remember a life-sized cuddly toy cat that somebody had given to one of the old ladies. Wherever she went the cat went too, finally out of the hospital altogether. In the grounds, however, the situation was different. The hospital was home to cats of all shapes, sizes and colours - although the dominant strain was small and black. It is easy to see why they caused alarm to infection-orientated minds, because they lived and bred in their own private warren, the networks of pipes and channels that criss crossed the grounds linking up the individual hospital buildings with each other and the boiler house, to distribute the hot steam which provided the central heating system. The pipes ran along narrow trenches, covered over with paving slabs, and out of the gaps and cracks in the paving, came the cats. During the day they occupied themselves cat-fashion around the grounds, taking care to keep out of the main thoroughfares, out of sight of people wearing white coats, communicating only at paws-length with those patients or staff-members with whom they were friendly, until tea-time saw each cat at its own kitchen door or curled up by its favourite radiator in the ward lounge.

CATS

SURPRISES

In the old days, when people spent long periods of time in hospitals like this, a great deal of effort used to go into providing entertainment for them, both in the main hall and in individual wards. Towards the end of the hospital's life a social centre for patients was opened in some old wooden huts that had previously housed a workshop for male residents, and people who could manage the journey were encouraged to go across there in the evenings to play bingo or to watch a different TV set from the one on their own ward. For those who were not able, too old or too ill to get across to the Patients' Centre, a group of people known as diversional therapists used to bring different kinds of entertainment to the various old people's wards - portable film shows, group games, quizzes and spelling bees, and, most important of all, the exchange of memories about 'how things used to be when we were young'. This last was to develop, eventually, into actual 'reminiscence theatre' once the Occupational Therapy Department was in full swing. That, however, came later. For the time being inward entertainment remained largely in the hands of the ward staff with the assistance of the patients themselves. Ward concerts were always rather unconventional, consisting typically of hymns and carols mixed with 'On Mother Kelly's Doorstep' and 'When Irish Eyes are Smiling', the whole accompanied by an itinerant ward pianist who was either a member of staff or a patient. Pianists were always appreciated and could depend on being kept busy endlessly performing on one or other of the dozen or so elderly patients' wards. These occasions were crude and unrehearsed; but what they lacked in skill they made up for in spontaneity and whole-heartedness.

SING IT AGAIN ...

Nice to be home again,
Lovely to get back.
It's a long day if you're not used to having people around you,
Even if they're your family.

Sally looked older, I thought.
I think she's missing John.
I looked at myself in the mirror, it's true, I thought, you do look younger,
Younger than my own kid sister.

Nice to be home again.
They're nice kids and it was lovely to see them.
Nice of them to invite me to stay until tomorrow.
They really made a fuss of me -
But this is my home.

This is my home now.
Twenty five years is long enough to get used to anywhere.
In twenty five years you really have time to belong,
To make your own world and live in it

NO PLACE LIKE HOME

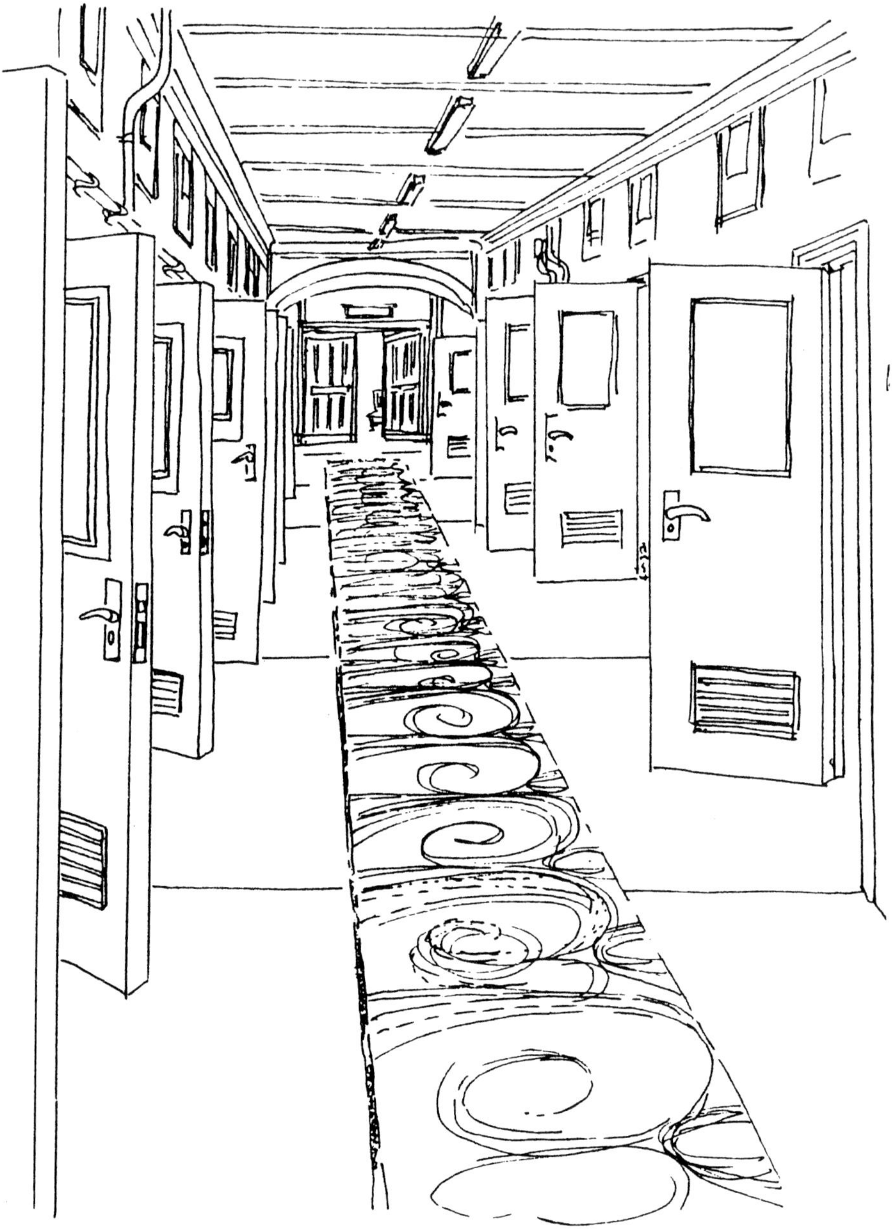

Tony had lived at Western Meads for a long time. An orphan, he had spent his childhood in a children's home where his closest emotional attachments were with children younger than himself. Later, when he reached his teens Tony was committed to the psychiatric hospital. There were few people of his age at the Meads: one other person left the orphanage at the same time, and bound for the same place. So far as personality went, Jane had little in common with Tony. Whereas he was quiet and withdrawn, tentative in his relationships with others, eager to please and anxious to avoid trouble, Jane had fiery red hair and a temperament to match. She was officially diagnosed as epileptic, but ward staff said she was only faking: it was temper, they said, not illness. She spent many days in seclusion as a way of calming her down ...

Tony's life at the Meads was happier than Jane's. Much of the time she was confined to the ward, he was outside in the grounds sweeping up leaves and lifting drain covers as part of his job with the hospital gardeners. This did not stop them finding each other, however. Divided within an institution that separated both from the outside world, Tony and Jane fell in love and made up their minds to get married. They were both over eighteen - just - and classified as 'informal' patients. Theoretically, at least, they were free to leave hospital and take up residence elsewhere. Theoretically, at least.

They did not receive much encouragement. It was more or less taken for granted that neither was in a position to contemplate anything like that. Nurses spoke of Jane's 'wildness' and Tony's 'dependent attitude'; doctors drew attention to the presence of epilepsy within the proposed marital dyad. It would obviously be unethical to sentence unborn children to life within a psychiatrically unstable environment - not to mention the disruption that would result in a place where any alteration in institutional procedures was out of the question. It seemed to go without saying that they were psychiatrically ill; why else would they be in hospital? They were used to being looked after, cared for. They must understand that they needed the kind of protection that only the hospital could give them. Had they any idea at all what it was like out there?

In spite of all this, Jane and Tony went ahead with their plans. The lady at the Citizens' Advice Bureau directed them to a lawyer, who said that they were legally free to marry. Next they approached the hospital chaplain, whom they both knew. This was a bit of a disappointment; it turned out that the hospital chapel was not licensed for weddings, so they would have to married at the Registry Office in town. Unlike the doctors, who continued to withhold their approval to the very end, the chaplain was won over by their obvious sincerity and strength and consistency of purpose - just the qualities they were supposed to be so deficient in, according to the hospital.

Once it was obvious that the wedding was going to take place, the hospital relented. If the marriage could not be prevented, it was to be encouraged! Arrangements were made for a reception on Jane's ward; staff and patients from all parts of the hospital came to church for the blessing service; people sent presents and messages of goodwill and collected enough money to pay for a brief honeymoon at a hotel in the neighbouring town. Sister herself gave Jane away at the ceremony and escorted them to the bedsitter which was to be their new home outside the gates. It was a wonderful day, one that we shall never forget.

FOR BETTER, FOR WORSE ...

The ladies on this ward, during the last fifteen years,
Constituted two groups: those who went out during the daytime
And those who didn't. If you yourself
Came into the ward not having been before
You might not have been able to tell the difference.
There's nothing special here. Just some elderly ladies
Sitting in armchairs, waiting for tea,
Not bothering to talk much.
You would probably have no idea, coming in like that from the outside,
Of the important class distinctions that hold sway
Affecting people's attitudes towards one another,
And the nursing staff towards each one of them.
You couldn't know how different from one another these people are:
Not a ward, but a world.

Three of these immediately classifiable people -
Typical psychogeriatric patients -
Have lived in this hospital since they were children.
Gertie, Ellen and Joan are called by their first names
As a sign of respect. They run the ward in co-operation with the nursing staff,
At the socio-cultural level. Mrs Andrews, however, sitting next to Gertie
Only arrived yesterday. She'll be here for two weeks
While her son and daughter-in-law are on holiday.

Gertie has a kind heart. After all, Mrs Andrews isn't a real resident.
Mrs White and Miss Townend, who are, both of whom
Having lived in this ward for a respectable number of years
Hold politely aloof.

LADIES ONLY

The really old part of the hospital is shaped like an H where the cross piece has been extended on both sides so that it resembles two plus signs joined together. While the outside of the building preserves an eighteenth century dignity and balance, its plan is strictly functional, conforming to nineteenth century scientific theories of social control. This is in fact the 'double panopticon' which is to be found in so many prisons and places of correction - and mental hospitals - built at this period and for many years afterwards. Once having taken up position at one of the points of intersection, whoever is in charge can look everywhere, keeping an eye on things north south east and west along the length of the four radiating corridors. Modern psychiatric nurses have never liked this arrangement. Apart from not being all that effective for 'ambulant' patients, it brings home the custodial role in a way that is nowadays felt to be unacceptable. This, however, is the architecture that they have inherited and must make the best of.

In later years, the line of sight has been interrupted by the erection of glazed partitions, which subdivide each corridor into distinctly separate wards, so that you would have had to pass through several other wards on the way to the one you wanted. At Christmas this could be a delightful journey, as each ward would be decorated in its own fashion by the patients and staff. The long central corridor, barrel-vaulted like the rest of the hospital, seemed like a succession of Aladdin's caves, each more fascinating and exotic than the one you were in and the journey developed from staging post to staging post, each new length of corridor a fresh unveiling - not at all what the architect had in mind.

KEEPING AN EYE ON THINGS ...

Come and sit down - have you got a few moments?
A few moments to have a chat? Go on,
You have. Sit down, that's right,
Next to me. Lovely! Now tell me,
How are you? How are you getting on?
Do you like it here? What do you think of the Day Hospital?
I love this place, you know. I do, I love it here,
Not like the ward. The Doctor said, try it, Pete, why don't you
Try it out! Give it a try! So I did,
And it's marvellous. Don't you think so?
People to talk to, things to do. Yesterday I even did a bit of dancing -
Plus a bit of acting. This morning I started on a coffee table
And painted my first picture since I was at school. Look, there, that one on the wall.
Sister put it there, she chose it specially out of all the rest ...
It was all right, nobody minded. You see, they're all
My friends, I've never had
So many friends, I really
Love it here.

I'LL JUST SIT HERE ...

Mary Collinge came to Western Meads Hospital when she was eight years old. She can still remember "when we were all together" - when she had been at home with her family for the first eight years of her life - but the memories were very vague. There seem to have been several siblings, plus someone called Auntie, but she could never remember the details. When, forty years after her entry into hospital, the hospital chaplain made enquiries on her behalf, no-one could be found. Even the Salvation Army 'family search' drew a blank. Nor was it clear why Mary had been admitted into hospital to begin with; at some time between nineteen-thirty-nine and nineteen-forty-five the hospital archives had fallen victim to enemy attack, and with them, Mary's past life up to coming into Western Meads. She was a mild woman, showing little or no signs of mental illness apart from the naive, childlike attitude to life that those who have spent a long time in hospital nearly always develop. The nurses described her as a happy patient, appreciated by almost everybody in the hospital for her friendly manner. The sadness in her life in hospital, the reason why she could be found wandering alone along the corridors, stemmed from her awareness of having been cheated of her birthright as a member of a family and made to spend all her days in hospital away from home.

Mary knew that she was in the wrong place, and spent her days waiting to be released. In the meantime she comforted herself by going to the hospital chapel whenever there was a service. The idea of being part of a family wide enough to encompass both the hospital community, where she lived, and the long-lost natural family, where she really belonged, seems to have appealed greatly to her. She talked about the chapel as if it were altogether different from the hospital in which it was situated; the hospital reminded her that she was a patient, the chapel that she was a person, a soul loved by God.

When the first group homes began to be set up, in the mid-nineteen eighties, Mary was chosen to be part of a group of patients sharing a house on a council estate about ten miles from the hospital. She was in two minds about going. She'd been at Western Meads for so long, she couldn't begin to imagine what it would be like living somewhere so very different. And what would she do about church? Fortunately, the hospital chaplain was on friendly terms with the vicar whose parish included the estate where the group home was situated. He suggested to her that she might like to start going to church when she left hospital, and described the church near the estate, and his friend the vicar. Mary took the idea up, and became a regular communicant at St. Cuthbert's. In fact, three out of four residents of the group home started to attend worship together.

This was the happiest time in Mary's life. At last she had a house of her own to look after and make into a home. She kept everything spotless, while making sure that the other three women fulfilled their household duties properly. Although shy, Mary was a genuinely friendly person. She used to invite the people she met at St. Cuthbert's back home to see the house. Anyone who dropped in to say hello was welcomed with open arms and given tea and cakes. Unfortunately it was a considerable walk to church, and Mary found it hard to get there by herself. There was talk of drawing up a list of people with cars who could give the group home ladies a lift on Sunday Morning. Before anything could be organised, however, one of Mary's companions had a serious stroke and had to be taken back to hospital. Mary reacted to the loss by throwing herself into the housework as if her life depended on it. When the social worker dropped in to see her she managed to preserve the impression that all was well, but her friends at church began to miss her when Sunday after Sunday she did not turn up for the Parish Communion. One of them called round to see her, and was alarmed by the excited way in which she was seized on and made to listen to all sorts of frantic plans for the future. Mary had been to see lawyers and estate agents, and had made steps to arrange a mortgage - unsuccessfully, because she had no income at all to spare and no prospects of having any. Her friend tried to remonstrate with her, wouldn't it be better if she tried to take things more calmly? Mary didn't listen, however. She simply went on from one outrageous scheme to another. Her friend tried to persuade her to seek help from the CPN*, but she simply laughed at her and told her not to be absurd, she was perfectly all right. Bewildered and frightened, Mary's friend reported the situation to Mary's doctor, and Mary was persuaded back into hospital for a few weeks.

This incident caused Mary's friend some heart-searching. She expected Mary to be angry and to say she had been betrayed. The Sunday after she was discharged, however, Mary was back in church again. She didn't refer to her stay in hospital except to say thanks, once, very quietly, to her friend.

All this was several years ago. Mary isn't able to get to church under own steam any more, and her friends at S. Cuthbert's have organized a rota for lifts on Sundays, and whenever there are socials and meetings of various groups to which she belongs: "She's always so appreciative. She has a wonderful effect on us all."

*Community Psychiatric Nurse

MARY

When Tom retired, as he was bound to do sooner or later,
We had the usual party for members of staff
And representatives of the RHA (Regional Health Authority).
Patients came too, although not specifically invited.
I'm delighted to see some patients here, Tom said.
I have many friends among the patients, he said.
And he was right. What nobody pointed out
Was that he had been getting on with them much better in his latter years
Since he stopped thinking about them as patients.
Never forget, he used to say to students and visitors,
Never forget these people are mentally ill. Don't go
Believing what they say.
At the ceremony, this patient said how much the patients appreciated all he'd done for them.
I hope he believed her.

GOING WITH THE FLOW ...

We grew all our own vegetables up on the hospital farm. Then we brought them down here, to the Vegetable Preparation Room. This was an old brick building, facing onto the builders' yard behind the cobbler's shop. It was a weird kind of place to work in, always full of steam - although the veggies weren't cooked there, only got ready to be cooked. It had great big garage doors on it, and when you went in it was like entering a huge cavern. They scraped all the potatoes by hand, using small knives, very sharp. If you cut yourself you'd have to drain all the water away, leaving the potatoes white and naked except where you'd stained them with your blood. Normally they floated in cold water, not in pans but in great big kettles, just like the kettledrums you see in orchestras. It was dark and cold and noisy. The noise in the Vegetable Preparation Room was different from anywhere else because the men who worked there permanently couldn't speak English very well. They were mainly from Poland or Lithuania or somewhere in that direction, and had come over as displaced persons. The place that they had eventually found was our Vegetable Preparation Room. The black glistening floor and the great bronze vats, the mixture of grease and polished metal, the steamy atmosphere and dim figures lurching backwards and forwards through it made the place feel like an old-fashioned railway station, even down to the embossed, green-painted machinery with its red lettering and brass handles: 'I speak your weight', 'Stamp yourself a name-tag', or 'See how much of a shock you can stand'. People stood about in groups. Nobody seemed to be doing much work ...

DISPLACED PERSONS

One thing about this place, it's always nice and warm
To come back to. When you open the ward door
The heat hits you. Hey I've brought you this, see,
I thought you'd like it. It's an icicle,
I'll put it in the sink for Sister shall I?
Here, let me sit by the radiator. I've done all my shopping
And most of Sister's. She tried to stop me going,
Said it was too cold, and that I'd slip and break a leg
Said I should behave my age. I said of course and what did she want
From the chemist's for her headache? She knows I always go,
Always into town on a Thursday. I always have
And always will. I've been doing it for forty years,
I'm not likely to pack it in now, am I?
Well do you think I am? Simply on account
Of a bit of weather?

COLD HANDS, WARM HEART ...

In the middle of the hospital is the huge recreation hall, used for all sorts of things - keep fit, badminton, workshops involving small groups, anything requiring space. Sometime, although less and less frequently during the hospitals latter years, there were brass band concerts and all sorts of visiting entertainments. Way back in the last century, when the hospital was famous because of its medical staff, the D'Oyly Carte Opera Company had performed one of the Savoy Operas here, on the fully equipped, professionally raked stage which takes up one end of the immense room. (Some say that Gilbert and Sullivan were themselves present on this occasion, but that may only be wishful thinking.) In later times, the stage was used for pantomimes performed by the staff and concerts given by troupes of amateur entertainers and local dancing schools. The hall itself is shaped like a huge oblong box. The ceiling is very high and quite flat, without any kind of protuberances. Even the stage was designed to intrude as little as possible; the main impression is of a large, deep cupboard entered by an ornately decorated archway and taking up no more than a third of the width available in the end wall. Sound rocketed off the stage and bounced back off the ceiling. The hall became an immense drum; it was full of sound and yet nothing could really be listened to, a state of affairs which made band music intolerable and any kind of stage performance impossible. For some reason, however, really big hospital occasions seemed to be improved by the throbbing noisiness of the hall. At gala dances held every Christmas and Easter, things reached such a pitch of excitement that the hall burst open with an irresistible impact, spilling out lights, streamers, and staff and patients in fancy dress - and noise.

LET THE TRUMPETS SOUND ...

I know I'll be all right if I just do
What Doctor said.
I must remember to try and always do
What Doctor said.
When I start to feel it coming on, all I have to do
Is what she said.
Hold tight, concentrate, think hard, I must do
What Doctor said.

I'd be all right now, if I could only remember what it was
Doctor said.

TRUST

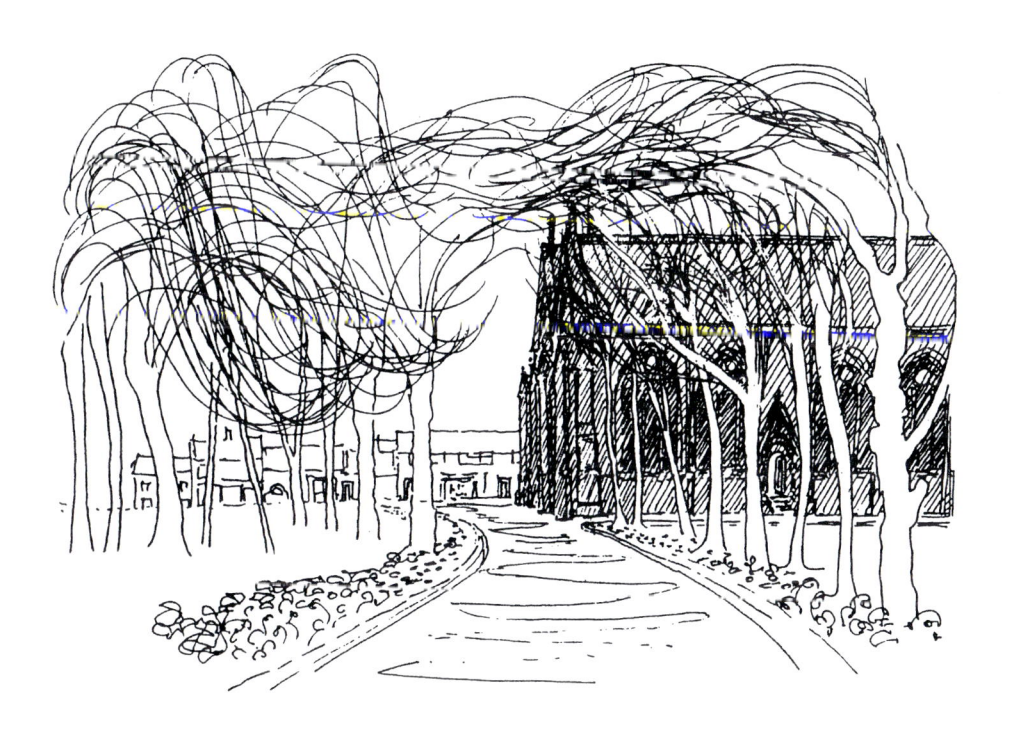

Here in Britain, nobody lives very far from some kind of church. Churches are social networks as well as places set aside for worship. Theoretically, at least, they provide opportunities for people who have spent their lives in institutions to make contact with existing social groups. Take the case of ex-psychiatric patients. Since the mental hospitals have started to close, many local churches in different parts of the country have found ways of helping former patients. Perhaps they welcome them into the various associations attached to the church. Sometime they co-operate with other churches to set up drop-in centres for people to meet and perhaps revive old friendships, because you need to keep hold of your sense of identity if you are to survive in an environment that is often, to say the least, not very friendly. On the other hand, this kind of involvement gives the church an opportunity to put its proclamation of love into practice.

Not everyone has responded, however. Local church leaders have said that, on balance, they would rather not commit themselves like this. Some say that the government should be doing this kind of thing, not they. It isn't the church's job to run the welfare state, they say. If the churches get involved at this level, the local authorities will simply say 'Over to you' and leave it to them. Behind these plausible-sounding arguments there is a fear of mentally ill people themselves, as people with special needs that no parish clergyman or congregation can possibly understand, never mind do anything about. That is the whole point of mental illness, people say: you can't understand it unless you're a specialist. This isn't necessarily the case, however.

George came to the hospital when he was sixteen, having spent his first years in an orphanage. He stayed for 36 years. His first Sunday at the hospital church the chaplain spotted him, thought he looked clean and cheerful, and asked him if he would like the job - unpaid, at least officially - as Server at the Communion Service. George did this for thirty years, under three successive chaplains, looking after almost everything to do with the church, both the building and the people who went there. He and the chaplain would visit the various wards in their blue cassocks, bringing comfort and reassurance to the patients. For many who lived there, George bridged the gap between patients and staff.

Now he lives on the other side of town, in a community of elderly people. He has been out of hospital for ten years now. If you talk to the other residents about him they will give you the impression of a man who is endlessly doing things for other people - collecting the groceries, doing the washing, helping dish out dinners, walking miles to carry messages, listening to people's worries and problems. He says that doing things for people is "my way of keeping out of mischief." He has always done things for people.

The difference is, now he's at liberty to do them. When he first left hospital he took his liberty to church, to see if it was needed there. It turned our that it wasn't, really. Folks were kind enough, but all the jobs had somehow been taken. He still goes, of course. In the meantime, the church's loss is the community's gain.

ENTER THEN HIS COURTS WITH PRAISE ...

Guide them with your Holy Spirit, Lord,
Wherever they may be.
Bless those living in the town,
The ones trying to make a go of it in hostels and group homes,
Help them to get along with one another and with themselves.

The happy ones, thrilled to be out of hospital,
In charge of something of their own at last,
Thank you for them.

And the lonely people, who miss their friends
And having something to do, and knowing
Where to go and whom to speak to.
Be with them, Lord.

People who exceed the quota of psychiatric beds
Allowed by the authorities for this area,
And can't get the help they need, for themselves and their families
Will you help them, Lord?

For all involved in and connected with these hospitals,
Those who have lived in them and helped to run them,
Those who built them for charity and those who have
Destroyed them for profit,
This prayer is offered.
And for ourselves,
We, who for one reason or another, have made Western Meads our home
Praise your holy name for the chance you gave us
To love and to care, to discover and to learn.
Lord, we praise your name
For the years we lived and worked together
In a place like that.

PRAYER IN A PLACE LIKE THAT

The chapel reflects the hospital it serves.

Hospitals like this are about separating people from people - and Gothic architecture is always useful if you want to keep people apart. The eminent architect who drew up the plans for the hospital chapel was well aware of this fact. He put it to good use by providing two parallel naves, each with a steeply pitched roof, like one of those old-fashioned railway stations in which the up line is separated from the down one by a row of cast-iron columns. Our columns were made of dressed stone, like the rest of the building, and they were there to keep the male and female patients from sitting next to each other in contravention of hospital regulations.

At some time during the next hundred years, it became clear to the staff that they no longer needed to exercise this degree of crowd control over the twenty or thirty women and men who now made their way across to the church on a Sunday morning. Now the congregation gathered all together in one place around the altar for a service very like Parish Communion in one of the churches 'outside'. As the group grew smaller its devotion increased. On important festivals, including their own Patronal Festival, the few remaining worshippers would process round the immense building, singing about their belief in Christ and their joy at being members of His Church.

At Christmas the people of St. Faith's used to hold a midnight Mass. The empty space on the disused side of the church became a stable, two members of the congregation dressing up as Mary and Joseph so that the others could sing carols around the crib. The custom lasted almost as long as the Hospital Church was to remain open; and patients from the new psychiatric ward at the nearby General Hospital, returning late from home leave, would notice the light on in the church and stumble in on half a dozen people singing away round an elderly Mary and a still older Joseph, while trying not to drop wax all over their carol sheets.

A CHRISTMAS CAROL ...

Tell me about yourself.
Strange how I start to drift when I hear people say that.
I suppose it's because it's not what I want,
You see. Without more information
I don't know what to do with it. They
Should tell me. They're the ones who are talking.
Why aren't they telling me anything, giving me some material,
Something to throw back at them,
Backwards and forwards, like a tennis ball. Tell me ...
About yourself; it's no good, I can't use it.
Perhaps one day I will, I'll let them know exactly who I am -
When I've more evidence to go on.

TELL ME ABOUT *YOURSELF* ...

The Gardeners' Department was situated in a small brick quadrangle, near to the Vegetable Preparation Room. Most of the time, of course, the gardeners were somewhere round about the grounds, mowing the lawns, weeding the huge flower beds, sweeping up leaves, rolling the playing fields. There always seemed to be a lot of them, and it was impossible to tell who was an employee from outside the hospital, and who a patient whose home was here, on one of the long-stay wards. The gardeners were very proud of their handiwork and would pause and share their pleasure with anyone with a moment to spare. They had every reason to feel proud; in summer their flowers surrounded the hospital with a penumbra of colour, like a dark stone in a summer garden. When it was really hot, the ward staff brought elderly men and women in geriatric chairs down in the lift and wheeled them onto the lawn where, among the flower beds, the emotional casualties of twentieth century living lay on the grass in their swimming costumes, sunbathing. When autumn came the gardeners loaded a wagon with flowers and vegetables and fastened it to the rear of the tractor to transport it along the gravel road to the hospital church for the Harvest Festival. This wide swathe of urban countryside belonged to the hospital patients. The space was not simply to separate two worlds but to give patients the chance to rest for a little between worlds. At Easter, the church was usually full of flowers and stood in the middle of a host of daffodils. On one occasion, however, the gardeners had forgotten and the congregation arrived to an empty church. Before the service began, one of the patients rushed in, her arms bursting with daffodils which she had obviously gathered from the ones around the church. After all, she said, it's our garden, isn't it?

OUR HOSPITAL, OUR GARDEN ...

Pad on left leg, grin on face
Derek goes out to bat.
It'll be some time before he's back.

The whites may not be very white
But the sun's as hot as ever.
It's a good way to celebrate your sixty-eighth birthday.

The other side isn't playing fair -
They've a couple of younger men playing for them,
Obviously members of staff.

Staff member or patient,
Mental hospital or village green,
The game is no respecter of persons.

At home on his own pitch,
An elderly man faces the opposition,
Hitting for six.

LAST MAN IN ...

As far back as most people can remember it was the usual policy to get as many patients as possible off the ward during normal daytime working hours, so that patients who were too old or too ill to be moved could be properly looked after. This means that most patients spent at least part of the day in some kind of environment designed to occupy their attention until the time came for them to go back to the ward. An important distinction was always recognised between patients who had no other address and people who were in hospital on a temporary basis, having their own homes to return to. The latter were directed to the occupational therapy department to spend their time in a constructive way doing things carefully designed to increase their interest in getting better and leaving hospital. The former weren't going anywhere and - generally speaking - knew it. All the same, efforts were made to provide the kind of work which, if not exactly interesting, would resemble life in normal social circumstances, by allowing them to earn a wage, albeit a very small one. Boring repetitive jobs done under contract for local firms - putting plastic animals in cereal packets, packing board games - brought in money for cigarettes and were the focus for social groups. Obviously this did not suit everyone, however; for one thing you needed reasonably agile fingers and serviceable eyesight. The elderly ladies and gentlemen on the 'old people's wards' would probably have liked to have stayed where they were once they had got up and had breakfast, but the habit of 'going to class' was far too entrenched in hospital practice; and besides, somewhere in the hospital there was always a working party, rudimentary in aim and limited in achievement, but where each person was regarded as a valuable member of the group and there was always someone genuinely glad that they'd made the effort to come along.

IT'S BETTER THAN BEING BORED, LOVE ...

The sparrow was rolling around on the ground, flapping its wings frantically. It was obviously in distress - "What's the matter with it, poor little perisher?" "Will it let you pick it up?" "Hey, wait a minute, there's something wrong with its legs. Look, it's only got one leg." "Oh what a shame, what'll it do?" "It's too late, it's dying." But the sparrow wasn't dying, as a matter of fact. It was only having a dust bath. It pushed itself up with its one remaining leg and took off, flying up into the air. Nothing wrong with its wings, you see.

If you saw Elsie walk across the room, you'd be very worried about her. She walks slowly, on the outside edges of her feet, swaying about as though she's going to topple over and fall. Sometimes she does fall, and you have to help her up again. But we let her walk by herself because that's what she wants. Elsie had a stroke and couldn't walk at all for four years. A couple of weeks ago she was still having to be pushed in a chair. But there's nothing wrong with her courage. When Elsie sways and totters, Elsie flies.

THE SPARROW

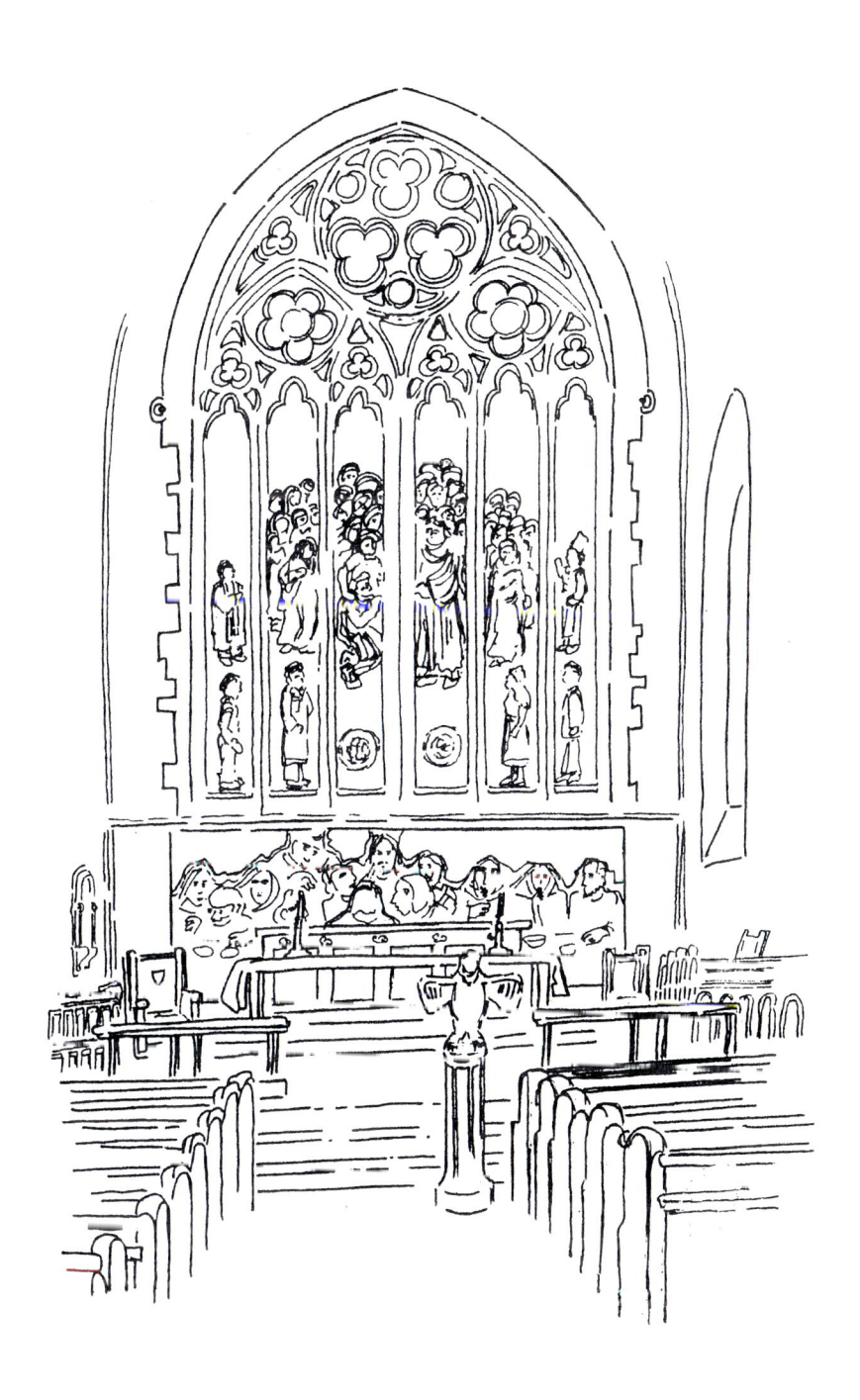

DIRECTIONS

It's a sea shore, you're kicking your feet through sand,
Warm, dry sand. Feel it?
Can you feel it?
There are stones now, round smooth stones,
Pebbles in the sand, can you feel them?
How does it feel? Suddenly sand again,
Warm and wet where the sun has warmed the spray ...
Do you feel it?

I feel something. Not sand. This isn't sand.
More like ground glass, but it doesn't hurt.
I can kick my feet through it as if it were sand.
Wait a bit, though -
It's getting clearer. Every second or third
Step, like a window in the sand
For you to look through. Hold on, perhaps
It'll come back again. No ... No,
It's gone. Beasts. Monsters. Like a kid's book.
This is what happens, I suppose
If you play kid's games. No, don't ask -
I didn't recognise anybody.
Well - not immediately ...

DRAMATHERAPY

Annette went to the hospital church every Sunday, except for the occasional weekends that she spent with her daughter and son-in-law, and those days when she felt too depressed to leave the ward. She always dressed neatly, with a smartness that was particularly welcome in hospital where it was so rare. She was both a divorcee and a widow, her husband having died a month after they were finally separated by law. Soon afterwards Annette came to Western Meads, where she was to live for nearly twenty-five years. Her daughter spent her childhood with her grandmother, her mother's mother. Now she has a husband and three sons - the family that Annette sometimes visits: "the children are very noisy, but I'm used to that, living where do,"

Annette is one of those patients who consciously adapted to the hospital. At some point she decided to make it her home, rejecting offers on the part of her daughter and son-in-law to give her a home with them. She stayed in hospital for years after her depression was controllable, making one or two close friends and being on friendly terms with everyone willing to be so, until the time came for her to be moved into the community, all these years later. She came as a voluntary patient, and left in the same fashion. She asked if she could have a flat, rather than share a group home or live in a hostel. Sociable without being gregarious she valued her personal space a great deal; she enjoyed the hospital because few people made claims on her, and she could move at her own speed with regard to the formation of relationships. For many years she wooed, and was wooed by, another patient, a man considerably older than her, whom she had known since she was a child; his family and hers were friends in the small local town they both came from. (Such hospital engagements seem to have been common at Western Meads. They rarely came to actual marriage, but were a great source of comfort.)

Annette left hospital six months before Trevor, who stayed on at the Meads spending most days wandering disconsolately in the grounds engaged in a symbolic search for his fiancée. Now and again she paid him a visit, but the move into her own flat made such a tremendous impact on her life that things belonging to the hospital began to lose their reality. She went once to see Trevor in the old people's home to which he was eventually transferred. She hasn't been since; the present is too interesting.

Her new flat is full of character and colour - plants, pictures, occasional tables, photographs of her daughter and grand-children, all her own things around her at last. A picture of her mother looks down from the wall: "She's smiling to see that I've my own house again at last." The change hasn't been all joy and celebration of newly discovered liberty; there have been times of extreme loneliness, sometimes of panic, when Annette realized the actual reality of isolation after so many years of being supported by the presence of other people. "If you cut your finger, and Nurse isn't there, and you don't know what to do..."

One of the things that has helped most is the link provided by her job in the packaging workshop that has been set up in the hospital grounds. Another even more important source of emotional comfort and practical help is the parish church, situated only a few yards away from Annette's front door. As soon as she moved in she started going to the family communion on Sunday morning. She seems to have settled in here without any difficulty; it is a very friendly church, and aware of the need to make strangers welcome. There are old links with Western Meads, particularly with the 'elderly severely mentally infirm' wards. The minibus from another parish church, which sponsors a drop-in club for ex-hospital patients, picks Annette up on Saturday nights and takes her back for an evening of coffee, conversation and bingo, For Annette, the Christian church has been crucial in easing the most difficult passage of all in a life full of drastic changes.

ANNETTE

The trouble with being a psychiatrist is
That one is expected to know everything
Because one is expected to know about knowing.

Certainly nobody expects us to be capable of everything,
Only to have mastered what capability is, in order to
Deal efficiently with incapability.

Why do I do this, Doctor? What have I got?
How can I stop doing it? Different kinds of question
Needing different kinds of answer.
Let's take the last one first. Yes,
I think I can stop you doing it. And if I can,
I can tell you what it is (or at least what we call it - and that's part of an answer to 'why'.
Not that I'm really convinced. 'How' is always
Easier than 'why',)

It can be lonely
When everybody thinks you know what's going on in their heads.
But when you yourself think so
It's not lonely enough.

HOW SHOULD I KNOW?

Vera was brought up in a village a few miles away from the hospital. Her mother and father were both churchgoers, and she used to go to Sunday School at the parish church every Sunday. She always enjoyed going to church and had happy memories of taking her own children to services: "We used to go as a family, me and Jack and the two little girls." The family lived close by Vera's own parents, and when Jack died - from a heart attack while still in his early forties - Vera was comforted and supported by them. She used to say that the double burden of grieving for Jack and feeling responsible for imposing this on two elderly people were the main cause of her breakdown and subsequent admission to Western Meads as a day patient. She was always extremely sensitive to whatever was going on around her. This worked both ways. For example, the birth of a granddaughter gave her a new lease of life, so that she was able to move into a flat on the local housing estate; on the other hand, the attitude of her neighbours on the estate upset her so much that she soon had to return to hospital on a whole-time basis: "She's one of those Western Meads zombies; they oughtn't to let them out!" This kind of remark made Vera particularly angry because of her intense loyalty to the hospital and gratitude for the help she said it had given her: "Nobody calls (i.e. insults) the Meads when I'm around!" During this second phase of her relationship with the hospital she made several close friends there, and kept in contact with them after leaving. She went to live in a single person's bungalow on a different council estate, her third home since finally leaving the Meads, the other two having been abandoned because of the hostility of the surrounding residents. Even here, she finds that people tend to be hostile and suspicious of ex-patients at the Meads: "They walk over my garden instead of keeping to the path, and if I say anything to them, it's 'Shut up and piss off, loonie.'" Vera has been free from any symptoms of illness for a year now. She realises that moving house is not the answer. Somehow, with the help of her friends from hospital she will survive: "After all, it's not anything to do with me personally. They don't know me at all, do they?"

COMMUNITY CARE

There's obviously been a change. These narrow rooms
With peep-holes in the heavy doors
Have completely altered their character.
Now they signify freedom, a kind of luxury,
A place of one's own at last.

At last, a room that is really mine,
Not shared with eleven other people
(I can remember when there were more than twenty.),
A proper dressing table, not just a locker,
And a heavy door.

The door is really weighty, resisting
People who push in to see me when I'm here
And want to be by myself, stopping
Thieves and intruders when I'm not in residence, protecting
Me and keeping me snug in my own world.

My own life. My room is where I keep my life.
I look through the peep-hole at you, at all of you,
And let you in or keep you out.
It's my choice.

A PLACE OF ONE'S OWN AT LAST ...

Ellen's funeral took place in the Abbey last week. It was quite well attended, mainly by members of the Abbey congregation, although a number of patients and staff members from the hospital went along to the service as well. Somebody commented on how surprised and delighted Ellen would have been if she could have seen the turn-out. Congregations are loyal to their members: she had been going to Sunday Choral Evensong for many years. A lot of people would miss her. All the same, she would never have expected them to take this much notice of her. Generally speaking, people didn't usually seem to consider her all that important. She had long-standing coolnesses with several ward sisters with whom, over the years, she had crossed swords, and she didn't see any reason why her reputation should be any higher outside than inside the hospital. Taken all in all, Ellen didn't think that much of herself. She was the kind of person who never asked much of life. In fact, she only wanted to be left alone to get on with her work. She was an extremely good worker, left to herself; but when Sister kept changing her mind, or wanted her to do either more or less than she was used to doing, she was liable to complain bitterly to anyone who would listen about the way in which she was being treated. It was amazing how angry anybody as placid as she was could become, once they were upset.

The fact was, of course, that Ellen was one of those patients who were taken advantage of from first putting a foot over the hospital threshold. It was so very easy to exploit a willingness to work which knew no bounds, representing as it did her end of a bargain she was quite willing to keep. The other end - the hospital's end - consisted in the understanding that she would be left alone to live her life in peace. She had come into hospital as a teenager. She was an orphan. The best efforts of the schools she had attended had not succeeded in getting her to learn how to read and write; that was not the kind of work she liked doing, and faced with the challenge of literacy she had retreated into her stubborn defence of her own privacy.

At the same time, Ellen liked people and enjoyed talking to them. She was not really as private a person as the nursing staff accused her of being. She talked rapidly, and her speech revealed the bizarre syntax that totally illiterate people sometimes make do with. She very rarely paused in what she was saying, as if she had never learned about sentences and full stops; and yet her meaning was clear enough, spurred on by her desire to communicate. So far as people in the hospital were concerned, Ellen was one of the folk who lived at the Meads as by right, almost as if they had been born there. It was her patch and she tended it with care. It would not really be true to say she was exploited - at least, not within the last twenty-five years of her life. The 1959 Mental Health Act saw the beginning of a movement to phase out the involvement of patients in the actual maintenance of psychiatric work. Up until then it was usual for such hospitals to employ patients as gardeners, upholsterers, painters, shoemakers, joiners, workers on the hospital farm and in the electrical and machine workshops. Despite its obvious openness to abuse - there were no union regulations concerning pay, for instance - the system had the advantage of giving patients a sense of being part of the actual running of the hospital. It was their hospital in a more real sense than it could ever be after the end of the sixties. Ellen, however, was permanently adjusted to this way of doing things, and when she retired from her jobs round about the hospital she took on domestic work for an ailing member of the medical staff, who treated her with a good deal of affection and respect, and was extremely grateful for the work she did for his family.

Doctor Dexter died. In her loneliness and grief Ellen turned to the Abbey, drawn by the splendour of the music and the beauty of the architecture; she had always been delighted by things that were done really well. The place obviously suited her. Something about the mixture of warmth and dignity, perhaps; the feeling of being left to yourself among people who are glad you're there: a privilege she earned a long time ago when she lived and worked at Western Meads.

REST IN PEACE, ELLEN

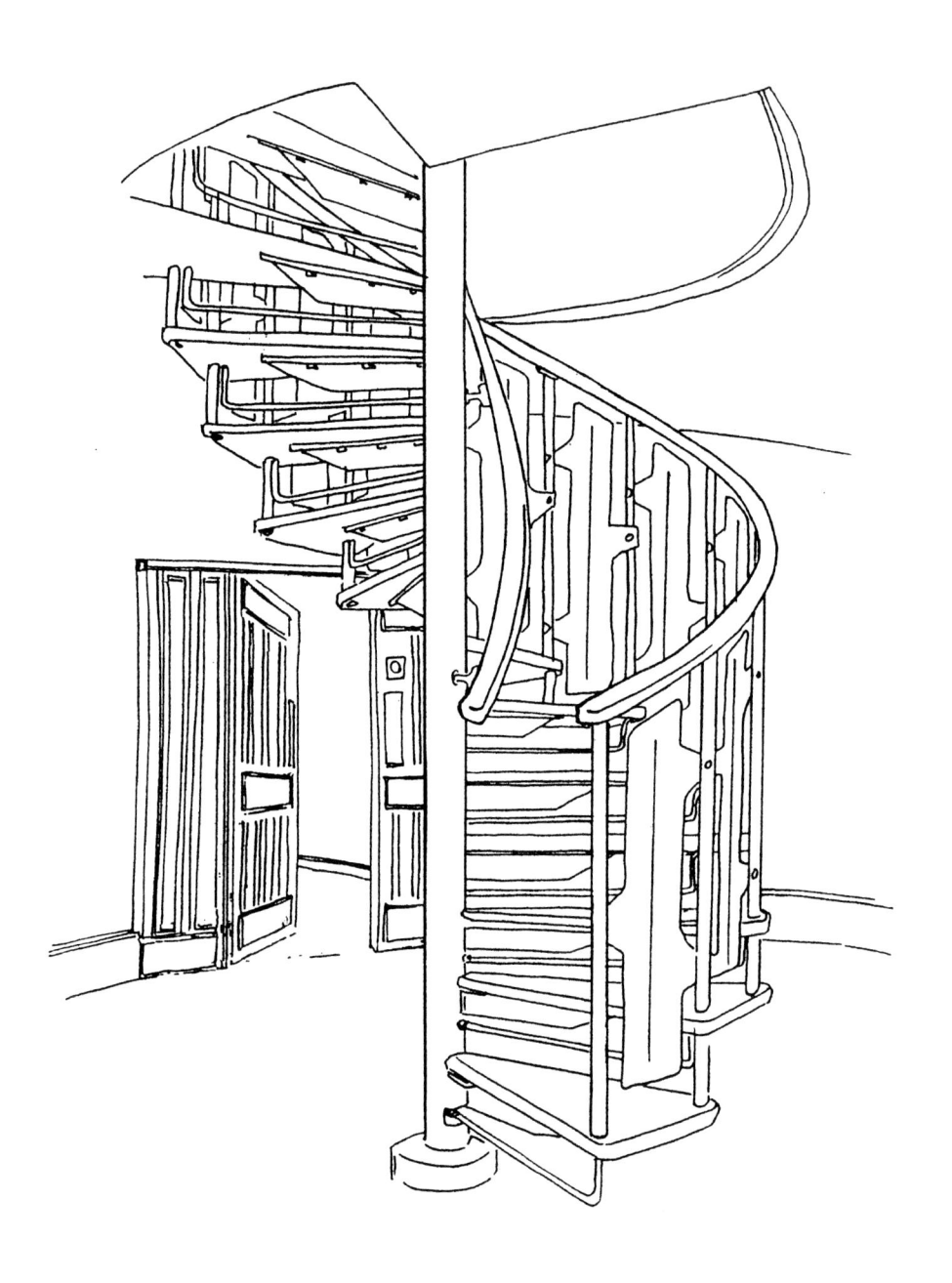

Wind-blown trees, small white clouds,
Nurses laughing and tumbling,
Reaching high to lasso the topmost branches,
Climbing on each other's shoulders
To hoist aloft a row of pennants. Sister stands
On tiptoe, to capture the highest twig.
One last stretch and maybe -
Skip - she's done it. Red, blue, orange, green,
Purple pennants dancing across the skyline,
Wreathing the distant hospital in bunting.
The NA's* run their streamers along the tops of the booths like Watteau's picnickers,
Running tiptoe through wrapping papers, cardboard boxes, tangled string,
Their skirts lifting at the hem, their hair blown high from their shoulders
Or whipping across their faces,
Half running, half dancing, bouncing, tumbling, clowning,
Seriously joyful.

* Nursing Assistants

NURSING SUMMER

Ted was born and brought up within a mile of Western Meads. In accordance with local custom the threat of admission played an important part in his upbringing: "If you don't behave, I'll have you put in that place!". Most of the time however Ted did behave. He worked hard at a local secondary modern school and did well enough in his exams to go on to teacher training college. Before finishing the course, however, he was offered the chance of going into business with an old friend, He took up the offer, and quit college for good. He was married and the father of a family when he found himself having to take Western Meads seriously again.

His first business venture had folded, and, after taking other jobs, he found himself redundant at the age of forty, with a wife, family and substantial mortgage to support. Ted always tended to blame himself for everything that went wrong; now his depression reached clinical proportions and he was admitted to one of the acute wards for treatment. After a few weeks as an in-patient, he began to attend the day hospital, and to take part in various kinds of group therapy. At this time a dramatherapy group had just begun to get under way, meeting for an hour a week. Ted had considerable experience as an amateur entertainer; he was delighted to find a suitable vehicle in which to express himself. "It really did me good, I was used to working in shows, but this was something different. No-one was competing, you see. It was about helping one another, not showing off." In fact this group worked together very well. The dramatherapy had been concerned with helping patients adjust to leaving hospital. Its effect seems to have been to direct members' attention to ways in which they might achieve some kind of continuity within the situation. Far from saying goodbye, the group members formed themselves into a social club which would go on meeting within the town after everybody had been discharged, carrying the friendship and support that people had discovered and enjoyed in the day hospital out into their ordinary lives. They decided to call it the Buffer Club - a reference to its function not to the age of its members....

There is no doubt that the idea for the Buffer Club originated with Ted, and that it was his enthusiasm and creativity that brought the club into being and developed its scope once the members had one by one severed their connections with Western Meads. The Buffer Club developed into the Initiative Group, which had the same membership but aimed to be more adventurous in its activities. It met - and still meets - every other week on Tuesday evenings.

The relationship between the Initiative Group and the neighbourhood churches is interesting. Ted and his family had been members of the Abbey congregation, a connection which went back into his childhood. When the Initiative Group was finding its feet, he and some of the other members paid a visit to the Diocesan Offices to see if the local church was interested in helping them with what they were trying to do - which at this time was mainly to keep going. They had heard of the existence of drop-in centres set up by local churches in a neighbouring town with a large hospital like Western Meads. The people at Church House provided them with a list of local parishes to which they might write. Three parishes replied expressing approval and promising support. As to anything actually happening, however, these parishes might just as well have done what the great majority did - which is, nothing at all. There were no meetings, no exchanges of ideas. The Initiative Group were profoundly shaken by this lack of response. Few of its members were churchgoers, but everybody had imagined that the church, if asked, would do something. Although he did not stop believing in God, Ted found himself less interested in going to the Abbey: "I think this is what God wants me to do. Obviously other people aren't so keen on doing anything. It's a pity about the church, though, isn't it?"

OUT ON YOUR OWN ...

Space isn't a problem, most of it's not used at all
Monday to Saturday, which means we've got
The time, too. Thursday? Wednesday? Friday evening?
It's really no problem And besides,
I'd like to do it. Somewhere for them to come, somewhere
Warm and friendly and cheerful, a place apart,
To meet old mates, so as not to lose with everything familiar
All at one blow....

What I have in mind is a kind of meeting-place
Cum talking shop. Of course, I don't know exactly what
They'd do - that's not up to me, they'll have to
Find that out themselves, I'm sure there'll be no problem;
The main thing
Is to have somewhere to do it. We'll do everything we can,

Premises, light and heat, transport for those who need it.
You see, there's really nothing to it. And besides
They don't want any fuss, do they? Strictly between ourselves
We've got a bar in the crypt, and a licence too,
Which I'm sure will be appreciated....

NO PROBLEM ...

The status of psychiatric patients has changed - officially, at least. Nowadays it is 'politically incorrect' to call them patients: the preferred term would be 'users of psychiatric services'. The various committees which represent interest groups involved in the provision of psychiatric treatment within the community (it's amazing how quickly you can pick up the language) usually contain representatives of 'user groups', it being generally agreed that those most personally involved in the treatment should have a say in determining the way in which the treatment will be administered (or, 'the service delivered'). In psychiatric circles this idea goes back to the attempts to set up special 'therapeutic communities' back in the 1960s. Nowadays, however, we tend to argue the other way round. In those days the idea was to create the kind of social environment within the hospital that was no longer available outside, except in rare cases where real neighbourhoods still existed. In those days, it was considered to be a matter of trying to establish the atmosphere of concern and acceptance that would have a healing effect on people who were psychologically wounded and socially rejected. Now we use 'community' in a different sense, to mean householders living lives that are financially independent: living 'in the community' simply means living 'outside the hospital'. The presence of users in the consultative process proclaims the equality and independence of every individual, their freedom to look after their own interests.

It doesn't work out like this, of course. Users and ex-users are not always able to argue their own case on committees, if the things they say cut across what are considered to be the interests of the non-users present. Being on such a committee doesn't do much for your self-respect. To be fair, however, it never did; even in the therapeutic communities of forty years ago, patients' councils were listened to but rarely obeyed. When it came to really important decisions about how the hospital should be run the cosmetic nature of user involvement was as obvious then as it is now.

Western Meads was an old-fashioned hospital. The Patients' Council only came into existence less than ten years go. Before that, the line between authority and dependency, patients and staff, was as rigidly drawn here as anywhere. One of the younger long-stay patients, who had been transferred to the Meads from a Home Office Special Hospital and was therefore used to a more rigid discipline and a deeper dependency than the regime at Western Meads, tried to set up a branch of what used to be called the 'Mental Patients' Union'. He made contact with other psychiatric hospitals in the North of England, and sent letters round the hospital to patients and staff on paper bearing the official union badge, a black spider's web and the letters MPU. Nobody really showed much interest, however, despite the hard work he put in trying to make the other patients as enthusiastic as he was. I remember him complaining to me that the younger ones were hoping for early discharge; they listened to him and agreed with what he was saying, but would really rather not become involved just at present. The older patients, those who had been at the Meads for a matter of years, tended simply to smile at him and say nothing at all. Today's Patients' Advocacy professionals will surely recognise the situation, sparing a thought for this pioneer of patients' rights.

THE SEMANTICS OF STIGMA

If you stand here you can see the whole hospital
Stretched out along the brow of the hill.
There are still a few patches of light showing:
Those over to the left are Mallison Ward
And the line in the centre is Denholme.
Otherwise nothing to show at all or very little.

It's sad to see it like this, isn't it. At this time of the evening
The hospital used to be a blaze of light. It's sad
To see it three quarters dark,
Almost completely dead.

LOOKING BACK

EPILOGUE: ASYLUM

Requiescat in pacem. Hospitals like Western Meads used to be called asylums. Places of refuge. Despite its modern connotations the name still has something of its old meaning. This hospital in particular retained an atmosphere of peace and rest. It was established at a time when mentally ill people were either kept prisoners in their own homes, shut up in attics or cellars, or exhibited publicly for the amusement of bored pleasure-seekers. During the first decades of existence, the hospital's rate of discharge was well up to modern standards. Certainly, this may be because the skill of psychiatric diagnosis was not highly developed and many people were admitted for what would now be regarded as mildly neurotic, or simply eccentric, behaviour.

The habit of regarding such hospitals as places of permanent, or semi-permanent, incarceration, repositories for unneeded lives, seems to have grown up around the period of the closure of the old workhouses at the end of the last century. The inmates were transferred to the local asylum, thus combining two kinds of social rejection, the fiscal and the medical, to produce a unique form of stigma. It was more difficult now to preserve the original idea of madness as an illness, and the hospital as a place of healing devoted to its cure. All sorts of unwanted people were admitted simply because they were unwanted; the hospital became a milieu for the living-out of inconvenient lives. Except for the period of the World Wars - when it seems a use could be found for everyone not actually incapacitated - the numbers rose steadily.

At every stage of its life, however, the hospital represented a caring response to human need. Founded at a time when such hospitals were genuine acts of faith in a compassionate God, a God of renewal and restoration, its stone buildings are the architectural embodiment of the urge not simply to contain and to master, but to heal. Towards the end of its life this original aim came nearer to fulfilment than it had ever been before, since the very first days of its life as a hospital. For the men and women who lived at the Meads during the last ten years of its existence there was more room, more personal attention than there had been in all those years of overcrowding, when a custodial regime aimed at suppressing all signs of individuality on the part of the unfortunate inmates, in order that the institution might function at all. During those latter years more effective control of the symptoms of illness made patients' lives much more tolerable, and encouraged the staff to treat them more like people than they were ever able to do before, Gentleness, concern, understanding, friendship, increased with freedom to share interests and ideas and to explore the experience of being human across the traditional barrier between patients and staff.

I myself noticed a great change taking place in the latter half of my time at the Meads. The focus of this revolution lay in the relationship between the patients and the nurses who looked after them. No longer were visiting students warned by the nursing staff that they should on no account take seriously any of the things they might be told by patients because "they are only patients'. In fact, in the last years of its life visitors to Western Meads frequently confused staff with patients, to the delight of all concerned.

It seems a pity that Western Meads should be closed down just as it was beginning to come back into its own as a place of genuine healing. The fellowship and sharing of insights and experiences that went on here among and between patients and staff would have brought joy to the hospital's founders as, at the end of its life Western Meads edged closer once again to the ideal of the Quaker missionaries from whose humanitarian vision it arose in the first place. The challenge that confronts us in the future, the success or failure of community care, can be seen at its most explicit - its most convicting - in the clear light of that original vision. Can we live up to it? Are we willing to bear the burden of trying? Isn't this our duty and joy?

I have written this book to express some of my own love for this hospital and to bear witness to the presence of love in the actions and words of the people who lived and worked here. I have tried to point to some of the many ways in which different kinds of human loving reflect their origin in the undifferentiated Love who is God. All the various kinds of human love are basically the same kind: the willing gift of the self to the other, and the reception of the other's answering gift in response. It is the change of circumstances that allows us to distinguish between them. Because we are creatures of circumstance, conditioned beings, we see change in everything that happens to us. Sometimes we see it where it does not really exist - or at least where its significance is secondary to things that have not, that will not, alter. We are so busy grieving over the state of the tree that we forget that there is joy and growth and life within the forest. Certainly, it is our tree, we love it, and we mourn to see the falling leaves. But it is our forest, too.

It is ours because it is God's and we are his. One of the most important things about the hospital was its situation. We were on a hill looking over the city, and from the top floors you could see the domes, towers and spires below, and the hills beyond. If you looked through the window of Willow Ward day-room, you were always conscious of a feeling of hope. Standing there looking out, it felt like flying. Down below were the palatial civic buildings along Forest Row, the parish churches, the magnificent spire of the Abbey. Between them and the hospital buildings were the trees, our own forest, surrounding the sports field and the hospital church, then marching up the hill, towards you. You were safe and free at the same time: safe yet free.

A lot of people need to feel this particular combination. Perhaps the whole human race longs like this. Security is not enough; we must have space to hope. It was a brilliant idea to build the new asylum on a hill within sight of the city, an even more brilliant one to put it in the middle of a forest. The wounded people who lived here wandered through the trees, and gazed over the town they would soon be well enough to venture out into again. Each found his or her own space to wander, his or her own particular vantage-point. Meanwhile the staff watched the seasons change in the forest, and the patients changing with the trees; drawing comfort and encouragement from the cycle of birth and death, giving thanks for reminders of things always known and continually forgotten. The hope that springs from despair, the kindness shown by people who have so much to bear themselves, yet find the strength to lighten another's load with a word or a smile, or some trivial action which shows respect for a fellow human being. Trivial had weight in a place like that.

Good-enough God. God who is good-enough for us. When we think of his love, we think of his Being, which means that we do not really think at all, but indulge in theological speculation. Sometimes we even think about Christ like this, drowning his humanity in a tide of wonder summoned up in our minds by the overpowering significance we attribute to his actions. We forget that Jesus is life-size, the right size for us. Jesus shows us that God is not only good but suitable. A more orthodox way of putting this would be to say that he came to make us suitable for God. More orthodox, but not more true. It works both ways, else not at all. In order to redeem men and women, God works through men and women with a skill which we can understand and appreciate although we do not always locate it correctly, and rarely expect it, preferring our own devices, our own ways of coping. I will not say that this does not matter; it certainly does. But it does not stop the God whose love is good-enough for even us to use. In all kinds of ways, he fits his love to our needs - not only the ones we know about but those we never imagined we had. At all times, and in all places, whatever happens to us, he provides us with what we need. Good-enough for his own Son, his love is ordinary and marvellous enough to wean us from our congenital human dependence into the glorious liberty of the children of God.

Rest in peace. This is how it was for me.
How it was, or how I saw it -
Observation, memory, sometimes only
Guesswork. A bit of a rush job really,
before the JCBs move in and there's nothing to build on.
Except rubble
And horror stories. The future will draw its conclusions,
Pronounce its own preferential verdict. All the same,
It has to be said, and should be recorded,
That there was goodness here as well as cruelty,
Love as well as fear ...

R.I.P.

1818-1996

The brain is a marvel,
The mind a mystery.

Sanity is a glimpse of sunlight,
Lunacy a probing of the Dark side of the Moon.

Madness and reason live together in us -
"Though this be madness, yet there's method in't."

The hurt mind trawls the depths, climbs the heights
of fantasy, and startles us with truth.

How then to contain, to save from further harm?
How then to honour the wisdom and foolishness,
The Truth in simplicity, the overwhelming sense of our humanity?
How to meet a social need, an individual sorrow, an impulse to care and heal?

In 1818
The strong walls came,
Not to exclude, but to give sanctuary.
The great gates swinging open, clanging to,
were there to shelter and protect
those inside, and those out.

Tuke, Ellis and Corsellis,
Ferrier, Crichton-Brown and Bevan-Lewis,
Bolton and their fellows,
brought wisdom, energy, enlightenment.
The Wards filled and extended.
From many causes, and in many conditions
the people came.
Driven by poverty, by social disgrace,
by illness and by fear.

Here was treatment, food and shelter,
A space to find your place in,
and that blessed word - Asylum.

Here was a Community, a world
where you might find a welcome,
succour, and some Peace,
and when the darkness came,
someone to hold
and to be held by.

Here was insight and ignorance,
Here was a struggle to be normal
in abnormal situations.

Work and achievement seen as healing arts,
Gardens and Farm, Laundry and Cobblers Shop.
A little town within a Town
Where the known things could be enjoyed,
and the unknown things contained.

Patients and staff. The Ward a family.
The staff the only mourners at a funeral.

Visiting relatives, spouses, children, friends,
bearing the silence, following the wanderings,
loving the inner friend, sitting and stroking,
holding on and letting go.

Laughing at Pantomimes, working light industry,
Alone in a corner, lost in your private world.
Fighting or quiescent, morose or driven by restlessness, depression
or unnatural energy.

Walking across the field to Church,
Groups from the Wards, Sunday morning,
Patients and nurses at one in the coming.
Candles and singing, the Gospel to greet us
and Johnny in his cassock.
The Bread taken and broken. 'Broken for you'.
'This is my Body broken for you'.
The hands, the eyes, devotion and life.
Lip smacking, murmurs of 'That was good.
Have you some more?'. Yes, we have more.
More than enough for patient and priest.
Joy in the sharing, joy in the being, joy in the morning.
Life, real life, here in this place.

Padlocks and notices. Fading farewells.
People on the move. Abandoned Victorian
tiles and solid mahogany.
The sense of the past, as well as the present
blessing the visitor, speaking quite clearly.
The trees in the grounds, the footballers shouting,
Conkers in autumn, paintings and cigarettes.
Times in the Tea Bar, sitting in sunshine,
Talking and happiness, silence and awkwardness.
Board Games and brightness in the Phoenix Centre,
- Life from the ashes.

Times change. Here the stones cry out.
Here is hallowed ground.
Here is pain and ease,
Order and disorder. Here is awash with tears
and such discovery.

Here shuffling steps and vacant stares
have changed to stillness and to open arms,
to a light in the eye and confidence
to put one foot before another,
to face the fear and speak your mind.

Here medicine has given independence
made life possible beyond the hospital gates.

Here neighbours and friends have found themselves again,
returned to homes and streets and families.
Here Gordian Knots of human entanglement
have not been cut, but gently straightened out.
Guilt and depression, self hate and violence,
The inner, deepest places, the common things writ large,
now brought into the light.
Here we have faced the fact that we can do nothing,
except to be there.

The skill of Consultant and of Counsellor,
Restraint and padded cell, baths and keys,
Drugs and skilled exploration of the human mind.
Time's healing, and a place as safe
and secure as we can make it.
Come and go, and welcome.

We celebrate the minds that thought of it,
The wisdom shown in guiding it.
Devotion, a hundred thousand acts of kindness,
insight, perseverance, battling for others, self-giving,
joyful and freeing, enfolding and life-giving.
Not us to them, or them to us, but the
daily discovery of belonging, of me in you,
and you in me, beyond the strangeness.
The brain is a marvel,
the mind a mystery .

Through our involvement here we have been blessed,
healed, restored. This is no place of mourning,
no place of ignorance. This is a place of honour,
thankfulness and life.
This is a place of Love.

Yes, that is it. The stones cry out of Love.
Crucified and risen. This is an Easter place,
of Cross and burial, and of Resurrection mornings.
Only the thousands who have been welcomed here
can know in themselves the great marvel,
the great mystery of Love revealed in this place.
Love has energised the work
and given it strength in all the healing arts.

The gates vanished - opening town to hospital.
Now the hospital has dispersed, fragmented,
moved elsewhere. We pray that everywhere the Love will grow,
remain, and find contemporary expression.
That those who come here now, - offices,
houses, will find among the stones that stay,
and the history of those that go,
among the mature trees, and the new building,
the same Peace on which they are founded.
The power in the Reredos, disciples' faces, intent,
and with great hunger for the Bread of Life.

On this 'Good Shepherd Sunday'
let us in our day know how
to Tend the Lambs and Feed the sheep,
to be good shepherds,
skilled in the ways of shepherding,
under the Good Shepherd of us all.

And when I pass this place,
or still walk about in it,
let the pricking tears,
the faster beating heart,
be the same as they have always been,
entering this lovely and loved place,
and all its people,
where I so often have come alive,
and left, to journey home
to a less vibrant world.

Ronald Ayres.
Written for the Thanksgiving Service at St. Faiths Church, Stanley Royd Hospital.   Sunday April 21st. 1996.

The West Riding Pauper Lunatic Asylum on East Moor is a very extensive and commodious building and from its extensive appearance, and internal management, is an ornament to the town and an honour to the Riding. It is under the control of the magistrates, and was founded by their order, under the authority of a general act of Parliament, passed in 1808 and amended in 1829; the cost of the land, building, furniture etc being paid out of the county rates, levied in the West Riding. It was opened in Nov. 1818, and considerably enlarged in 1830 by the erection of a new wing, and other offices - the number of the unfortunate inmates being, in 1836, no fewer than 173 males, and 148 females, mostly paupers, sent hither by the warrants of magistrates under the provisions of the act, which requires that all pauper lunatics and dangerous idiots, shall be sent to such institutions and that the weekly payment of 6s. for the maintenance of each shall be paid out of the poor rates of their respective parishes. C. C. Corsellis M. D. is the resident physician; J. Bennet and S. Marshall are the surgeons; and the Rev. N. J. Naylor is the chaplain.

William White. History, Gazetteer and Directory of the West Riding of Yorkshire, 1836.

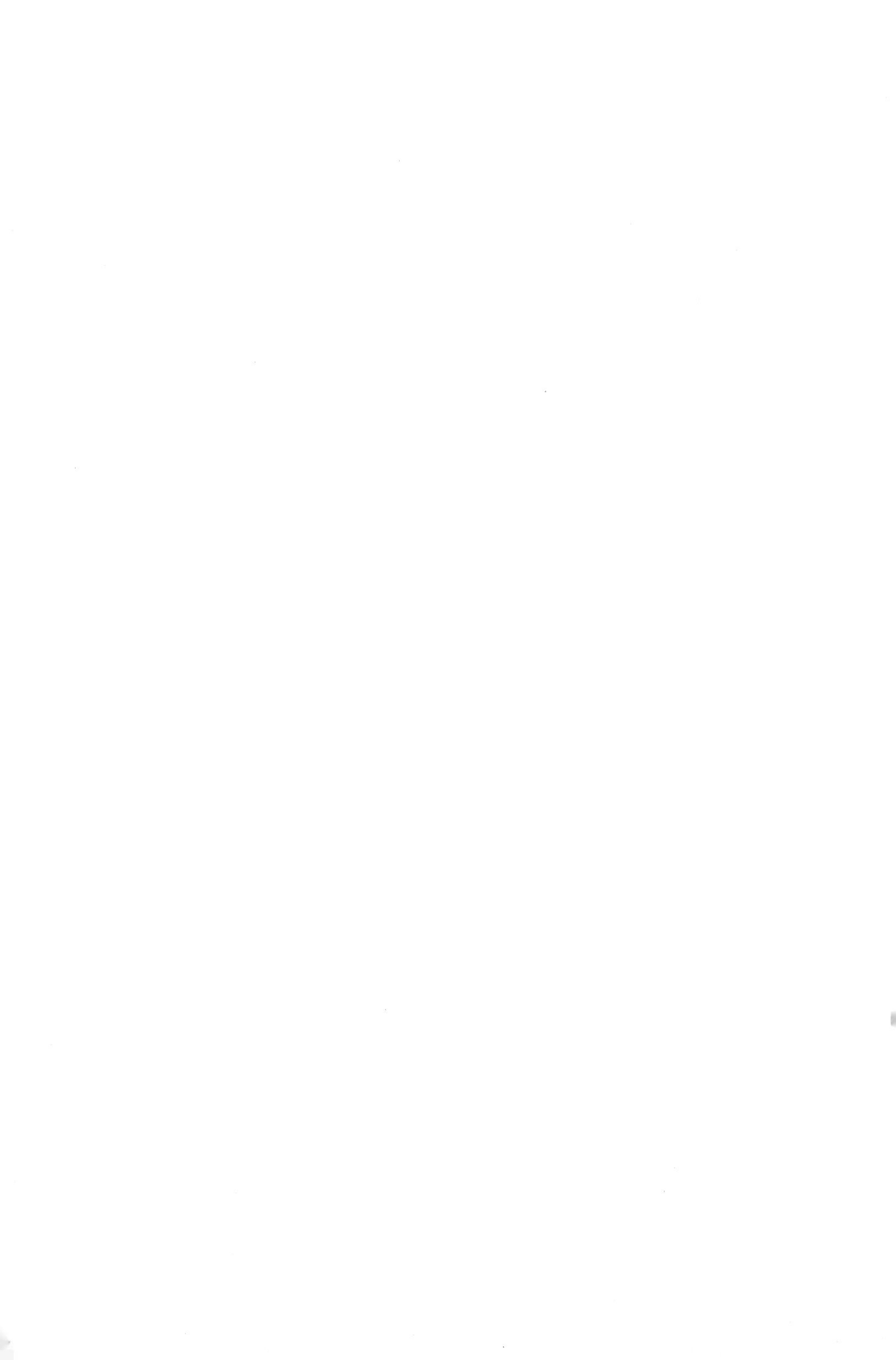